ASK YOURSELF:

- Do you become anxious when you think about going to the dentist?
- Do you cancel or fail to keep your dental appointments?
- Do your palms feel sweaty when you walk into a dental office?
- Does your heart begin to pound rapidly when you get a shot?
- Are you hesitant to smile because your teeth look bad?
- Do you notice that you have bad breath but cannot force yourself to visit a dentist to have your teeth cleaned?
- Do you postpone dental treatment that you know you really need?
- Do you think your career or your relationships are being hindered by the current condition of your mouth?

If one or more of these questions applies to you, you may be suffering needlessly from dental fear or dental phobia. You should know that you have the right to have a healthy mouth, a beautiful smile, and the freedom to visit a dentist comfortably. Read about how you can discover information that can make a significant change in your life.

"What also impressed me was the fact that this is one self-help book that really provides a lot of self-help. Many books cross my desk every week on health topics of every kind, and many of them promote themselves as self-help books when they really are too shallow or preachy to do any good. This book lets patients learn about their fears, identify them, think about them, write them down and do something to overcome them. For fearful patients, that's what's really important. They already know what the consequences of their fears are; what they need is help."

- Sue MacDonald, Health Columnist, *The Cincinnati Enquirer*

WHAT AN EX-FEARFUL
DENTAL PATIENT HAS TO SAY

This patient, for many years, postponed extensive dental work because she had several fears regarding dentistry. She was referred to our office and she went through our dental fear self-help program. She then, over a period of several months, had her dental treatment successfully completed. She did extremely well throughout this lengthy treatment and, being well satisfied, wrote the following letter to our office to share her feelings with us.

"Dear Dr. Bob,

Words could never express how grateful I am to you, Dr. Bob, for my newly acquired dental work and bright smile. I could never have done it without you, your fear control program and your beautiful staff. I love you all.

I had so much apprehension about receiving the dental work that I so very much needed. I can't believe that you were able to take me through all the procedures. Your dental work is beautiful. I am very proud.

You are a very dedicated professional and I admire all the hard work you put into it. You are so enthusiastic about helping others. Truly you are one of God's special people.

May you enjoy continued success in all you do.

In appreciation,

Mrs. X"

Letters such as these really "make our day." Seeing a fearful patient become relaxed and have his or her dental treatment successfully completed is a great reward for my staff and me as well as for the many other dental offices who render dental care gently and compassionately.

If you have been postponing dental work that you know you really need and want, you owe it to yourself to find out how this can happen for you.

HOW TO OVERCOME FEAR OF DENTISTRY

DISCOVER HOW PROVEN METHODS
CAN HELP YOU OVERCOME
BARRIERS TO ORAL HEALTH
AND A BEATUTIFUL SMILE

HOW TO OVERCOME FEAR OF DENTISTRY

Robert F. Kroeger, D.D.S.

Private Practice of General Dentistry
Cincinnati, Ohio
Lecturer, Department of Oral Health Science
College of Dentistry, University of Kentucky
Lexington, Kentucky

HERITAGE COMMUNICATIONS

CINCINNATI

Library of Congress Cataloging-in-Publication Data

Kroeger, Robert F., 1946-
      How to overcome fear of dentistry.

        Bibliography: p.
        1. Dentistry — Psychological aspects. 2. Fear.
I. Title.
RK53.K76 1988   617.6'001'9   87-82919
ISBN 0-9618291-1-7

Published by:

Heritage Communications
11469 Lippelman Rd.
Cincinnati, OH 45246

10 9 8 7 6 5 4 3 2 1
Printed in the United States of America

Cover and illustrations by Creative Dimensions, Cincinnati.

CONTENTS

This book is dedicated

to the millions of dental phobics

in this country and in the world.

I hope that this book may offer

them encouragement and promise and I hope

that this book may also elevate, in their eyes,

the image of dentistry as a

trusted and caring profession.

FOREWORD

As a boy who grew up with lots of cavities in the era of the low-speed dental drill, I suffered pain which at times seemed as if it would never end. As a result, I became tense and anxious in the dental chair well into adulthood, despite the fact that modern techniques had reduced real pain to a minimum.

As a psychologist, I learned that my lasting tension and anxiety were part of a natural conditioning or learning process which can be reversed; dental fear (or phobia) can be unlearned. Unfortunately for the fearful patient, the process does not always occur in the natural course of events. It may require a special effort under appropriate conditions. Now, fortunately for that patient, Dr. Kroeger has laid out those conditions and described in detail methods by which dental fear can be overcome.

The techniques described in this book are based on sound psychological principles and each has been shown to be effective in the reduction of a wide variety of human fears and phobias. The many cases cited by Dr. Kroeger

testify to the fact that dental fears are no exception and that
he is among the pioneers in the application of these techniques to dentistry.

Inclusion of these methods in dental school teaching is
relatively recent, but more and more dental students are
being trained to deal with extremely fearful patients. For
example, this year I incorporated Dr. Kroeger's book, *Managing the Apprehensive Dental Patient,* and his tapes into the
behavioral sciences course at the Harvard School of Dental
Medicine. Someday, every dentist will be highly skilled in
these special methods for reducing dental fears. Until then,
if you are a victim of this problem, you may need to seek out
the special sources of help listed in this book. But, whether
or not you require special professional help, reducing your
fear will require some effort on your part. Useful as it is to
read about and understand the psychology of your fear, in
order to overcome it, you will have to expend effort in
learning systematic relaxation and in using it to desensitize
your fear of dentistry. Dr. Kroeger has described the methods; now it's up to you to put in the effort. The potential
benefits are worthwhile and extend well beyond having your
teeth repaired. They can lead to improved appearance,
greater self-confidence, and a generalized improvement in
your ability to handle stress.

Gerry Kress, Ph.D.
Director of Educational Research
Harvard School of Dental Medicine

PREFACE

I have written this book to help the millions of individuals who feel uncomfortable during their dental visits or who completely avoid visiting the dentist. Writing this book has been a long-term goal for me. In accomplishing this goal, I have learned many useful concepts and techniques that have helped me in my personal life and in my dental practice. I hope to pass these on to you, the reader.

Years ago, in practicing dentistry, I noted that extremely fearful patients often would seek my care only for emergencies — a toothache or broken filling. After their emergency was treated, they would not return for a complete exam. In 1982, I designed the dental fear control program, a self-help, non-drug approach to overcoming fear of dentistry. In 1985, I did a research study of over 100 patients who had participated in this program. The results of this study were encouraging. Almost 100 percent of the patients said the program helped them to overcome their fear. Seventy percent said that if they had not gone through the program, they probably would not have returned for treatment. This confirmed my experience that fearful patients often seek only emergency care because they do not know how to deal with the fear barrier.

Many patients who do visit a dentist on a regular basis also have tension and anxiety, to some degree, during their dental visits. This book is intended to help these patients as well as those who are too fearful to make regular checkup appointments. The book may also help the dentist and staff understand dental fear from the patient's point of view.

Many dental phobics think that having their dental work completed under general anesthesia (being put to sleep) is the only way possible for them. They should realize the risk factors of general anesthesia. They also should realize that the fear barrier is not eliminated with this mode of treatment.

Patients who do not have *regular dental care* usually, over a period of years, develop serious dental problems such as extensive decay and gum disease. The idea behind this book is to allow the patient to uncover his or her dental fears, cope with them, and learn effective ways to relax in the dental chair so that dental treatment can be successfully completed.

Although I personally have devoted much time and effort to writing this book, I would like to thank all those other people who helped and supported me: all my fearful and phobic patients who stimulated me in this direction; my entire office staff of receptionists, hygienists, dental fear control therapists, and dental assistants who, over the years, have shown me that these principles work effectively.

Thanks also go to the faculty of the University of Kentucky College of Dentistry, especially Dr. Tim Smith and Dr. Ray Mullins, for their support, encouragement, and guidance; to Dr. Gerry Kress of Harvard University for his support and for teaching these concepts to his dental students; and to Drs. Weinstein and Milgrom of the University of Washington for their research efforts that helped me apply these concepts to dental practice.

I am grateful to all those who helped me assemble this information from rough drafts into the finished book. These suppport people include proofreaders: my sister, Mary Beth Dunn, my parents, Mr. and Mrs. Frank Kroeger, and Mrs. Lynn Lipson. I would like to thank Anne Montague for her content and copy editing and Ion and Amy Itescu of Seven Hills Books for their many contributions to help make this book a polished gem. I would like to thank all those reviewers who contributed many useful ideas: Sue MacDonald, Dr. Gordon Rubin, Dr. Tim Smith, Dr. Hal Forman, Dr. Bill Wathen, and Dr. Enrique Kaufman.

I would also like to warmly thank my wife, Brenda, for her patience and commitment, including caring for our young children — Kimberly, Robby, Jonathan, David, and Michael. I deeply appreciate their support, love, and tolerant understanding.

Many case studies of fearful dental patients are presented. Although the examples represent actual patients, names have been changed to insure confidentiality.

1

INTRODUCTION TO
FEAR CONTROL CONCEPTS

Dental fear affects about 75 percent of the U.S. population to some degree. Fear makes people cancel or simply not show up for dental appointments. Their teeth can get worse and their gums can become diseased. About 10 to 15 percent of the population has dental phobia, a condition that causes complete avoidance of dentistry. This can result in abscesses, infections, oral cancer, and other problems that can harm one's general health.

Take this self-quiz to see whether you have dental fear or dental phobia. Answer yes or no to each question.

1. When you think of having an oral injection or having drilling performed, does your heart begin to pound rapidly?
2. Do you have a specific fear about some aspect of dentistry that you feel you can never overcome?
3. When you think of visiting the dentist, do you remember a bad experience you once had and again feel your heart

pounding?
4. Do you frequently cancel or fail to keep dental appointments for a variety of reasons?
5. Do you try to rationalize why you cannot afford the dental work you know you really need?
6. Is everybody in your family afraid of dentists?
7. When you walk into a dental office, do the smell and the noise make you feel uneasy?
8. At your last appointment, did you have one of the following: sweaty palms, pounding heart, nausea, tense feeling in general?
9. Would you like to be put to sleep to have all your dentistry done?

If you have answered yes to one or two of these questions, you will benefit from this book. If you have answered yes to several, you will be helped by this book but you will probably also need the dentist or a psychotherapist to work with you in special ways to overcome your fear.

WHAT IS FEAR?

Fear, as defined by Webster, is an unpleasant, often strong, emotion caused by anticipation or awareness of danger.

Dental fear is an unpleasant emotion that causes a patient to have apprehension about dentistry. It may cause patients to cancel appointments or put off treatment. It may cause a patient to have an uneasy stomach or sweaty palms during the visit. Dental fear can cause people to neglect their mouths, resulting in a large bill for restoration of the teeth. Routine dentistry is not expensive. Neglect is expensive. Dental fear, if it grows, can become dental phobia.

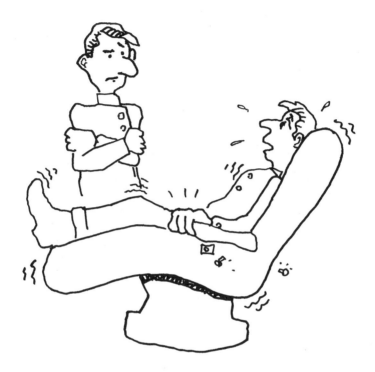

"Dr. Jones, would you like to cancel this appointment?"

WHAT IS A PHOBIA?

A phobia, as defined by Webster, is an exaggerated, usually illogical, fear of something.

Dental phobia is an intense fear of dentistry, exaggerated to the point where the patient completely avoids visiting the dentist. Many dental phobics would almost rather die than visit a dentist. They are experts at treating and medicating themselves. This almost always compounds their initial problems. About 8 to 15 percent of the U.S. population has dental phobia. This means that 25 million to 40 million Americans avoid the dentist completely because they have this problem.

FEAR VS. PHOBIA

Fear is derived from the Middle English word *faer,* meaning sudden danger. Fear is a normal response and can be lifesaving. It consists of three components. The first is an unpleasant state of mind, such as a feeling of impending disaster. The second is behavioral: shaking, restlessness, and an attempt to avoid the danger. The third component is the physiological stress response: sweaty palms, pounding heart, muscle tension.

A phobia is a fear that has ballooned out of proportion, interfering with a person's daily activities. A phobia can be described as an unreasonable or an irrational fear of something. It can be fear of an object, situation, place, or one's own internal reactions. Phobias are much more paralyzing than fears and usually cause avoidance behavior. While fear sometimes can be beneficial (if you're being attacked by a grizzly bear, you need fear to energize your body to run for safety), phobias are burdensome, disrupting one's career and social relationships.

A child who is locked in a closet for punishment by his or her parents may develop claustrophobia, an intense fear of being confined. As an adult visiting the dentist, this patient may feel uncomfortable in a tiny treatment room, especially if the door is closed and the room has no windows. This same claustrophobic patient may feel smothered by the facial mask for nitrous oxide sedation (laughing gas).

Fear is a learned behavior. But whatever is learned can be unlearned. You can conquer your dental fear or dental phobia. The first step is to realize that it is your responsibility to overcome your fear. Many a fearful patient has placed himself or herself in the dental chair with the expectation that the dentist must do it all. The fact is that the dentist and staff cannot do it all. The patient can contribute *greatly* to reducing his or her fear level and making it easier for the dentist and staff to deliver gentle dental care. This book is aimed at showing you, the patient, both how to overcome fearful behavior and how to select a gentle dentist.

I myself used to avoid dentists at all costs. I've had the same fears and the same concerns that many of you have had. Let me tell you my story.

When I was a young boy (probably about four or five years old), I went to a dentist who was rather harsh. This dentist never gave me any novocaine when he drilled my teeth. I can remember vividly the pain I endured. I recall the very slow, pulley-driven drill, the dental assistant holding me forcibly in the chair, and the tears running down my face. I had several sessions with that dentist. He died when I was about ten.

The new dentist my family selected was compassionate enough to use novocaine to numb my teeth before he drilled. However, by that time, I was sensitized to dental pain. I expected to have pain when I heard the sound of the drill. And I always did have pain during drilling. Perhaps this was because I was conditioned to experience pain when I had drilling done. Perhaps it was that this dentist never waited long enough for the novocaine to numb my teeth because he had only one treatment room. But I was a smart little fellow. I knew I would have pain during the drilling, so I tried to create a greater pain to distract myself: I would pinch the skin on my thighs as tightly as I could to produce intense pain in my legs to distract my attention away from the pain in my teeth. That worked well enough to help me endure those treatments.

We can learn some things from my childhood experience in the fifties. First of all, dentistry was much different then from what it is today. Like everything else, dentistry has grown, learning from researchers and scientists. Local anesthetics are much more effective today in preventing pain. When I have a patient who raises his or her hand indicating pain, I can apply additional numbing agents to stop the pain. Then the patient is pain-free during the drilling nearly 99 percent of the time. Even ten years ago, I could not make that statement.

Secondly, we can see that even though I was given a local anesthetic, novocaine, I still had intense pain during drilling. This may have been because the dentist did not wait long enough for the anesthetic to become effective. Or I may have been so conditioned to dental pain that the novocaine could not work well. Many people think that they will *always* experience pain during drilling, no matter how much novocaine they are given. Some think they are immune to novocaine. The more likely explanation is pain conditioning related to some type of a bad experience. In the next chapter I will explain thoroughly these concepts pertaining to pain perception. It is extremely important to understand these principles. They demonstrate why fearful or phobic individuals are more likely to have pain than those who are not fearful or phobic.

By overcoming dental fear and having your mouth and teeth restored to health, you should realize the following benefits:

- An increase in overall health, since the mouth directly and indirectly influences one's health in general. Decayed teeth and gum disease harbor many harmful germs that can cause serious infections.
- An increase in career opportunities. Did you ever see a salesman smile with a mouthful of broken and discolored teeth? What effect does this have on the potential sale? A smile has a powerful persuasive effect.
- An increase in social relationships. Would you want to kiss someone who had a mouthful of decayed teeth and diseased gums? Today communicable diseases are more prevalent than ever before.

- An increase in self-esteem. When you overcome your dental fear, you will experience a strong sense of accomplishment, and rightfully so. And being able to smile with a beautiful set of teeth gives many patients a huge boost in self-worth. Life becomes fun again.
- An appreciation of good dentistry. Many patients do not appreciate the value of fine dental care. The fearful patient, once he or she learns that he can have his mouth restored gently and comfortably, will value his investment in excellent dentistry for the rest of his life.
- A reduced cost per dental visit. Extremely fearful patients require more dentist and staff time than non-fearful patients to accomplish the same procedure. This extra time results in a higher bill.

My goals in writing this book are the following:

1. To help patients help themselves overcome fear of dentistry.
2. To help patients feel comfortable enough to return for regular checkup visits.
3. To help fearful patients eliminate the habit of canceling or missing dental appointments.

What are your goals? What do you hope to accomplish after finishing this book? Your best bet is to think about the following suggestions and then write down on a piece of paper your goals regarding your mouth and your health in general. Tape this paper to your bathroom mirror and look at it several times each day. This technique, together with an action plan to carry out your goals, will help you reach them.

Goal 1   To overcome my fear or phobia of dentistry.
Goal 2   To select a dentist to help me achieve excellent oral health.
Goal 3   To make, keep, and be on time for my dental appointments. To have a support person help me, if necessary.

Goal 4   To follow through with the necessary dental treat-
          ment to give my mouth the care that I deserve.

Goal 5   To develop a warm and friendly relationship with
          my dentist, dental hygienist, and dental assistant.

Goal 6   To practice excellent oral hygiene, as recom-
          mended by my dentist, including the use of den-
          tal floss daily. To also monitor my intake of sugar
          and other harmful foods that may damage my
          mouth and teeth.

Goal 7   To return for my checkup visits on a regular basis
          as suggested by my dentist or hygienist to main-
          tain the dental health that I have achieved.

Now, after thinking about what you really want, write
down your goals on paper and place this paper where you
will review it daily.

2

SOURCES OF DENTAL FEAR
AND DENTAL PHOBIA

What is the basis for fear? Lack of understanding? Lack of confidence in a situation? A Pavlov-type response?

Pavlov was a Russian scientist who experimented with evoking a response from animals. He used a dog for his famous experiment. Pavlov simultaneously flashed a light and gave food to the dog. He did this repeatedly. He discovered that the dog would salivate whenever this happened. Eventually, the dog, anticipating food, would salivate whenever the lights were flashed, even when no food was present. The dog had been *conditioned* to salivate by associating the flashing lights with food.

Many dental phobics are similarly *conditioned;* they experience an array of physical and emotional symptoms (pounding heart, sweaty palms, thick saliva, stomach butterflies, nausea, increased blood pressure, shortness of breath, dizziness) in response to a number of stimuli (white walls and white uniforms, the sound of the drill, the sight of a needle, the smell of a dental office). Figure 1 illustrates these symptoms. If a patient suffers intense pain during drilling, the sound of the drill will bring the expectation of pain. Many former dental phobics enjoy using stereo headphones to block out the sound of the drilling to lessen the effect of this conditioned response.

Over the years, other experiments have demonstrated that fears are acquired and learned, typically through personal experiences but also through the media and hearsay.

THE CIRCLE OF FEAR

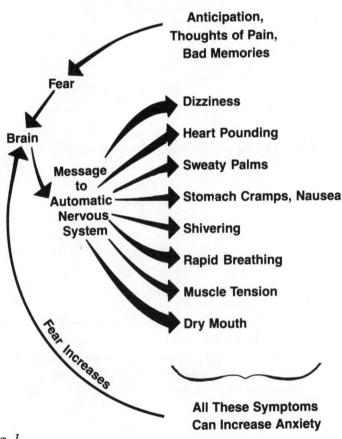

Fig. 1

Consider the various ways dental fear or dental phobia is acquired. As you read each item, ask yourself whether it applies to you. Try to understand where your fear originated. Identify your fear or fears. Later in the book, treatment strategies will be presented to help you to deal with a specific fear. But the first step is to identify the source.

PERSONAL EXPERIENCE

Bad personal experiences play a dominant role in generating dental fear or phobia. Children who have never been hurt in a dental office are much more cooperative than children with bad dental experiences. Studies have shown that past experiences of fearful patients contribute significantly to the origin of dental fear or phobia.

The Hospital Experience

A person can become fearful of physicians, dentists, and needles through a negative experience in a hospital. A young child (or an adult, for that matter) with an injury may have to wait in the emergency room for hours before he or she is treated. And what does he see and hear while he waits? Painful, fearful expressions, people crying, and people in acute distress. He notices that everyone in charge (physicians, nurses, and other staff) are dressed in white uniforms. He notices the white walls, white sheets, white towels. An association is recorded in his memory bank connecting injury, pain, and fear with white walls and uniforms. If the child or adult also suffers a painful experience in this hospital environment, this negative association becomes even more firmly fixed.

When the child or the phobic adult patient walks into a dental office with white walls and finds all the staff and dentist dressed in white, what goes through his or her mind? The prior bad hospital experience is flashed back and intensifies the fear or phobic reaction. Many dental staffs wear colored uniforms to eliminate or reduce the possibility of triggering the memory bank. Also, some hospitals are trying to change their image by adding color to their walls and uniforms, as well as by adopting a caring attitude.

An example of an injury-generated phobia is that of Eric, age 25, who had a phobia centered on blood. His phobia is the result of a car accident that left him covered with blood. Then he was operated on in a hospital where he again remembered being covered with blood on occasion. Afterwards, he would faint at the thought or the sight of blood. Soon after this experience, he consulted a psychiatrist but did not follow through with treatment. He fainted once when he saw blood on the sidewalk.

Eric's needed extractions of several hopeless teeth and extensive restorative procedures. We decided to try to keep him from seeing any blood. He agreed to go ahead with this plan.

Unfortunately, before some simple procedures could be done to help alleviate his phobia, he developed a toothache from several decayed teeth that were to be extracted. The teeth were removed surgically, some bleeding occurred but was controlled, and the appointment went smoothly. He used headphones and nitrous oxide sedation. After the appointment, as he stood at the front desk, an alert assistant noticed that he looked pale. She escorted him to a chair and summoned me, because he said he was going to faint. Soon after I arrived, he fainted. After reviving him, we took him to a treatment room for oxygen and for time to rest. Several minutes later, he again went to the front desk area, where again he said he felt faint. He was escorted promptly back into the treatment room, where he again fainted. Finally feeling well rested, he left the office in a cab.

We felt we did a good job with Eric's treatment, but probably underestimated the severity of his phobia. I called him later that evening and learned that he was very happy with our treatment and, in fact, said that it was the easiest dental visit he had in his life. I was surprised at that comment.

Eric has returned for further treatment. At each visit, his fear is reduced. He is very excited about having his mouth restored. He recently sat through a two-and-a-half-hour procedure and left in good condition. He has not fainted since the initial visit.

The Medical Office Experience

Another factor in instilling fear is a bad experience in a physician's office. Fear of needles can begin after a rough, careless injection or blood-drawing from a vein. Often, the first contact a child has with the field of medical care takes place in a pediatrician's office. If poorly performed, the normal childhood immunizations can be a source of fear of needles and, again, of white uniforms.

An Injury to the Teeth or to the Face

A serious injury of this type can sensitize the patient to further work around the face or mouth. A disfiguring car accident, for example, can result in a lesser self-image, especially if a self-image problem already exists.

The loss of a tooth, especially at an early age, can be psychologically troubling. Sometimes, males may feel some loss of virility when they must lose a tooth. Patients having had teeth knocked out, incisor teeth fractured, or associated cuts to the mouth will do very well if their injury is treated gently, compassionately, and efficiently. However, this treatment usually involves an injection to the front of the mouth which, for a young child, can be upsetting.

The Negative Childhood Dental Experience

A bad childhood experience in a dental office can create a phobia that is probably the most difficult psychological block to overcome. In childhood, first impressions form vivid images and build lifelong memories and attitudes. Some dental schools and experts still recommend the hand- or towel-over-mouth technique: The dentist places his or her hand or towel over a child's mouth until the child cooperates. Most dentists today do not use such techniques. Rather than resorting to physical abuse, the dentist can halt the procedure, place a temporary filling, and refer the child to a pediatric dentist who specializes in treating only children.

Karen, one of the patients who inspired me to do extensive research to develop the dental fear control program (see Chapter 5), came to my office several years ago with an abscessed lower molar. This was her first visit to a dentist in ten years. Karen was a pleasant 26-year-old who appeared normal psychologically, except for her dental phobia. She was crying when I met her.

When I asked her why she felt so fearful, she said that as a young girl she was treated by a dentist who was her uncle and who regarded her as being pampered. (She did not appear this way to me.) During one appointment with him, she began crying because she had pain during the drilling. At this, the dentist told her, "Shut up." When she continued to cry, he slapped her. That is the last thing about the treatment procedure she remembered. As she was taken to her parents in the reception room, she regained consciousness. Her face was covered with black and blue marks and blood. After that, she seldom went to a dentist.

Karen did well in our office, responding to gentle care. With the use of nitrous oxide sedation, she managed to have her treatment completed.

This is an example of how a bad experience can traumatize a child and sow the seeds of phobia. Karen may never

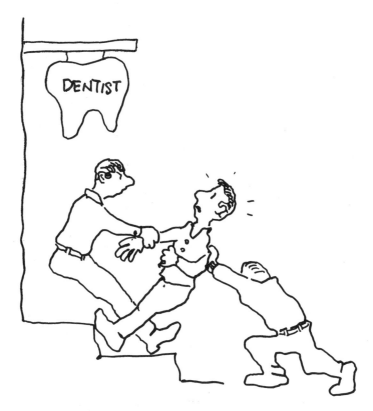

"Actually, I think aspirin will take care of my toothache."

forget the painful past but she looks forward to the future and deeply desires to save her teeth.

Fearful and phobic adults often report that, as children, they received minimal dental care because their parents could not afford proper care. This treatment often involved painful injections or extractions at a school clinic. Today, it is sad to see a young child being presented to the dentist with badly decayed baby teeth, even worse with a toothache, on the initial visit. The child's imagination often will magnify the pain or the bad experience into something worse than it actually is.

The Negative Adult Dental Experience

Adults can usually reason and understand concepts better than children. However, when an adult sits in a dental chair and reclines into a vulnerable position, he or she places a certain trust in the dentist and staff. If this trust is abused, a great distrust and fear of the dentist will develop. A patient with a bad experience as an adult usually has an easier time overcoming his or her fear or phobia and responding to fear conrol therapy than an adult who had a bad dental experience in childhood.

Some adult experiences, however, can be particularly painful. Valerie, a 50-year-old homemaker and businesswoman, had not been seen by a dentist in 15 years. Her dental phobia stemmed from a bad experience in an army dental clinic.

At that time, she was seven months pregnant. She reported to the clinic, in pain, with an abscessed tooth. She was told she could not have local anesthetic for the procedure. On a flat examination table, Valerie was held down by four people while the abscess on the roof of her mouth was lanced. This excruciating pain initiated labor and delivery of the baby (six weeks early). Valerie did not want to discuss this experience in detail and was uncomfortable remembering it. She also had other experiences of being assaulted in the head and face.

Her first visit, after the fear control program, involved a cleaning under nitrous oxide sedation. She did well, had her treatment completed, and thrived on guided imagery (described in Chapter 4) for relaxation.

Lifestyle and Attitude

Some patients have difficulty accepting the authority of a dentist or of any other person. Some people never grow up. Pampered children often develop the attitude that the world revolves around them. In adulthood, these people may not change much. They are frequent complainers and exhibit a negative attitude toward life when they face the reality that they are no longer the center of attention. A definite correlation seems to exist between this type of attitude and the source of dental fear. This person often arrives with a toothache and uses hostility to mask his or her fear, resulting in a bad experience for both patient and staff. This person is usually demanding and finds it difficult to accept concern and caring from the dentist and staff.

George was this type of patient. He arrived in my office with a dental emergency — two badly decayed upper molars. My staff reported he was rude and unfriendly during the interviewing process. As I talked with George, I noticed his eyes never left his lap. This indicated extreme distrust and low self-esteem.

He told me that many dentists and physicians in the past had told him he would not be hurt, but he always felt much pain during treatment. He didn't think this visit would be any different. I told him his hostility was shielding his fear, and this fearful behavior was reinforced by other dentists who told him to disregard the pain he was feeling. I told him successful dental treatment is a two-way street; he must give me cooperation and I would do my best to be painless. I explained that sometimes he might feel pain and, if this should occur, he should signal me to stop. Despite this detailed and concerned explanation, he still would not look at me. I then began treatment with novocaine. The deep decay was removed and temporary fillings were placed. I stopped when he signaled that he was in pain. At the end of treatment I did not think he would return. However, as I was walking out of the treatment room, I heard George say, with a wide grin, "Thanks, Doc, you were great."

George did return the next week for examination. He related that he grew up in a rough neighborhood and reported being kicked in the head and face area in several incidents. And he told me about several bad dental visits, including one when the dentist placed his knee on George's chest during a difficult extraction.

George took the dental fear control program, and afterward his trust level began to build. During several visits, he had deep decay removed *without pain* while only novocaine was used. At each visit, George managed a wide smile before he left.

George's phobia, when unmanaged, made him feel more pain. After he began to successfully manage his phobia, he had no pain under similar circumstances. In the next chapter, you can see why a dental phobic can experience more pain than someone who is not fearful.

A Poor Self-Image

For one reason or another, some people have a poor self-image. They are usually negative thinkers and believe in an external locus of control, such as fate or luck. They are firm believers in Murphy's law: If something can go wrong, it will. Poor self-image may be a cause of a fearful attitude toward the dentist. It takes a certain amount of courage and self-confidence to recline into a vulnerable position in a dental chair. Those who have a poor self-image may lack this confidence and may allow this phobia to increase significantly and keep them away from the dental office for a long time.

A Poor Oral Condition

Here, a snowballing effect may occur. The diseased oral condition of many fearful patients interacts with any bad experiences to increase the fear or phobia level. This type of patient becomes more fearful as his or her oral condition worsens. He feels ashamed to show his mouth to anyone, and imagines the dentist or staff will criticize him severely for allowing his mouth to deteriorate so badly. He imagines the dentist and staff will make fun of him. He also worries that a tremendous amount of dental treatment may be required.

NONPERSONAL EXPERIENCE

The Media

Nonpersonal experiences can also influence the way a person perceives dentistry. These can reinforce a person's fear or phobia. Probably the most damaging nonpersonal cause of dental fear is the powerful influence of radio, television, newspapers, magazines, and books. Everyone who watches television or reads is exposed to jokes about dentistry. Usually they refer to pain, fear, or fees. The writers of these jokes are looking for a good laugh, of course. But, in actuality, they are reinforcing the image of dentistry as painful and expensive. This image is unfair and deceptive. Quality dentistry, although involving an initial investment, will endure the test of time and be a better economic value than low-quality dentistry. Negative images in the media increase the fear level of millions of patients and rekindle painful memories of fear-producing experiences. This may drive people further away. The resultant deterioration of the diseased state of their mouths can lead to complete loss of teeth, oral cancer, cases of serious swelling, and even death.

A few years ago, an ad promoting a computer system appeared in a national magazine. It said learning to understand most computer systems is as painful as having a root canal performed. An astute endodontist (root canal specialist) wrote a letter to the computer company saying he and every dentist he could influence would boycott the company's products. He also wrote a letter to the *ADA News,* which is read by tens of thousands of dentists and dental staffs nationwide.

The Marathon Man is an example of a movie depicting dental torture. An ex-Nazi dentist is shown drilling without any novocaine into the nerve of a live tooth of his victim to obtain information. Many fearful and phobic patients become nauseated when watching such a scene, feeling they are reliving their own bad experiences.

What can people do about this negative media influence? Anyone who cares can write to the journalist, author, or performer to inform him or her of the harm he or she is doing by emphasizing the painful image of dentistry. This may help eventually to change the painful and fearful image of dentistry that the media perpetuate.

Hearsay from Friends and Relatives

Stories and exaggerations told by others can make patients refuse certain types of treatment. As a child, one is influenced first by parents and siblings and then, as a teen-ager, by friends and classmates. Individuals who tell stories about their own dental experiences may persist in this behavior because of an age-old concept that misery loves company.

Recently, I saw a 34-year-old patient who was extremely fearful of dentists. Dave had seen a dentist who told him that he had periodontal (gum) disease and that he probably should consult a specialist (a periodontist) for surgery. Dave was afraid of this treatment but did return to his general dentist for visits every six months. He told me that he dreaded each visit and was relieved when the visit was finished.

Dave said he could not remember any personal bad experiences involving dentistry. However, he did say that he had heard a lot of rumors about dentistry that influenced him. These horror stories from his friends and his relatives made him apprehensive enough to postpone his needed treatment. Dave will need corrective gum surgery, which is not a pleasant thought for him. First, though, he must overcome his fear — the reason for his avoidance of dental care. He will go through the dental fear control program and he will be desensitized in our office. When his fear is controlled, he will then be ready to see a periodontist who will help Dave save his teeth. Unfortunately, because of his procrastination over the years, some of Dave's teeth will be lost because of bone loss associated with his gum disease.

Cultural Attitudes

In certain subcultures, negative attitudes toward dentistry are formed that are difficult to change. These attitudes portray the dental visit as painful and costly. Many people are influenced by these attitudes before they ever visit a dentist. They are often surprised that a tooth can be saved instead of extracted. These attitudes convince people it is natural to lose teeth and wear dentures. Sometimes fearful attitudes are transferred to children by parents who tell children to be brave and not worry about a dental visit. I once met a seven-year-old who wanted his badly decayed baby teeth extracted so that he could wear dentures as his parents did. Many people choose to spend money on television sets, vacations, and other "necessities" while neglecting their oral health, claiming dental care is too expensive. Numerous other attitudes exist that have a negative influence on a person's dental experience. Often, the dentist can erase these erroneous beliefs with a rational explanation of the facts.

Several years ago, a patient of mine needed root canal therapy but refused it because her family convinced her that it was painful and a waste of money. Despite a detailed explanation, the patient again refused, trusting the dubious advice of her relatives. This attitude prevailed throughout the entire family, including aunts and uncles.

In some parts of this country, the idea that dentures are

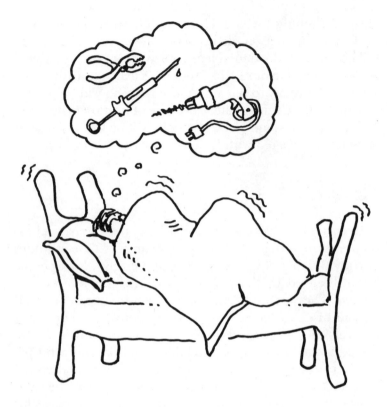

The night before "The Appointment."

inevitable is prevalent. This type of mental block makes it very difficult for the dentist to convince patients that they can save their teeth for the rest of their lives.

SEVERITY OF YOUR DENTAL FEAR OR PHOBIA

In addition to knowing the source of your dental fear, understanding the severity of your fear or phobia may also be helpful. Moderately fearful patients and dental phobics are usually in a state of acute distress prior to a dental visit. This distress period can range from a few hours to a few weeks preceding the appointment. This produces the physiological signs (see Figure 1) of a pounding heart, sweaty palms, dry mouth, muscle tension, and difficulty in breathing. Behaviorally, the patient may be irritable, act impulsively, laugh nervously, appear restless and trembling, and have difficulty speaking. Psychologically he or she may feel frustrated, moody, threatened, and guilty, and eventually develop low self-esteem. Many dental phobics are ashamed of their mouth and feel very childlike in their fears. The patient may be hypersensitive to criticism, or forgetful, and may have trouble making decisions. One can see why some dental phobics, in acute distress, will cancel, fail to keep, or be late for dental appointments. (However, once desensitized by a caring dentist and staff, the phobic is usually very punctual for appointments.) Phobic patients usually arrive at the dental office in this state of disarray, often trembling and in tears.

To identify patients as being fearful or phobic is very useful for the dentist and staff. The fearful patient is easier to manage and requires less counseling time than the dental phobic. To help categorize fearful and phobic dental patients, I described the following classification system in a journal called *General Dentistry*. It is reprinted here with permission.

Fear Level One

A patient at fear level one will exhibit typical signs of the physiological fear response during a dental appointment. However, this patient visits the dentist on a regular basis in order to prevent the consequences of neglecting his or her mouth. Usually he responds well to a compassionate "chairside manner" on the part of the dentist and staff. The fear control program is offered to these patients, but normally they do not feel they need it. They are manageable during the dental procedure and may respond well to nitrous oxide sedation. They may not enjoy their dental visits and they may exhibit some anxiety throughout the session. This type of patient would benefit from the fear control program and, after taking the program, would probably not become anxious in anticipation of a dental appointment.

Fear Level Two

Here, fear intensifies and causes the patient to avoid the dental office. A patient at fear level two does not visit the dentist on a regular basis for preventive maintenance. This patient will go to the dental office only if he or she is in pain or has a dental emergency. He may have had a painful experience in dentistry or medicine that causes his fear. He may also be under acute stress from his personal life, job, or social situation. Although a gentle, compassionate "chairside manner" may help this patient get through the emergency procedure, this will not usually be sufficient to motivate the patient to return for an examination and definitive treatment. The dental fear control program works well to help this type of patient overcome his fear enough to have his dental treatment completed.

Phobia Level One

This level represents a patient whose fear has intensified beyond fear level two, resulting in more severe avoidance behavior. This patient will do everything he or she can to avoid the dental office, even if he is in pain. He may be skilled in home remedies and may have avoided the dentist for five to ten years or longer. This patient often has a deteriorated mouth with rampant decay, abscesses, and gum disease. Upon questioning by the dentist, the patient will admit he avoided seeking dental care, even during extreme pain. Again, remember what a phobia is: an *unreasonable or irrational* fear.

So what motivates this patient to seek dental care? Sometimes, he will arrive with a dental emergency or a toothache, usually with swelling. Occasionally, he needs to be hospitalized because of massive swelling that has invaded his face and neck. Often, however, after years of encouragement by a trusted friend or relative, the patient will make a decision to seek a dentist's help. This decision usually is based on assurances that the dentist and staff will be kind, gentle, and noncriticizing.

This type of patient will not respond to merely a compassionate "chairside manner." However, the dental fear control program works well in encouraging this patient to accept needed treatment.

Phobia Level Two

A patient at phobia level two exhibits the same avoidance behavior. However, in addition to dental phobia, he or she may have other significant psychological problems related or unrelated to his dental phobia. He often comes with a specific problem and, once treated, does not return for additional treatment. Usually his behavior and speech patterns reflect an irrational and unpredictable thought process. His appearance may be unkempt or meticulous. He may use psychological "games" to mask his fears. His fear may be manifested as hostility.

Usually, the person's self-esteem is low. He may make statements like, "Life is going nowhere for me" or "I feel depressed often." Sometimes, a person may be obsessed about a particular aspect of dentistry. His obsessive neurosis is better handled by psychotherapy. Also, a very phobic individual who does not accept or respond well to the fear control program and refuses sedation may be a candidate for psychotherapy.

A patient at this second level of phobia usually does not respond well to the fear control program and would benefit from treatment by a psychologist or a psychiatrist. A referral to an appropriate professional should be made by the dentist.

	Physiological Fear Response	Seeks Regular Care	Motivated By Pain To Seek Care	Responds To Fear Control Program	Additional Significant Psychological Problems	Time Since Last Dental Visit ψ
Fear Level I	Yes	Yes	Yes	Yes	No	Annual
Fear Level II	Yes	No	Yes	Yes	No	2-4 Years
Phobia Level I	Yes	No	No	Yes	No	Over 5 Yrs.
Phobia Level II	Yes	No	No	No	Yes	Over 5 Yrs.

ψ - The time since a person's last dental visit is a general, not a specific indicator of fear/phobia type.

Fig. 2 - Summarizes the categories of dental fear and dental phobia.

SELF-ASSESSMENT

At this time, you should have a good idea of the source and severity of your fear or phobia. Try to complete this self-test as accurately as you can. By discussing these items with a friend or with your dentist, you will start the process of overcoming your fear of dentistry.

A. Source of my fear or phobia

1. Did I ever have a bad experience in a hospital or in a medical office?
2. Did I ever have a serious accident involving injury to my face or teeth?
3. Did I ever have a bad childhood or adult experience with the dentist?
4. Do I have trouble accepting authority?

5. Do I think I know it all?
6. Do I act with hostility to people I don't know?
7. Do I feel that I have little self-confidence in many situations?
8. Do I feel that my mouth is in awful shape? Do I feel that this is increasing my fear of dentists?
9. Do I become apprehensive when I hear or see something on TV, radio, magazine, or the newspaper that highlights the painful image of dentistry?
10. Do stories or talk from my friends and relatives make me uneasy about going to the dentist?
11. Does my family have the attitude that dentists are painful and very expensive and teeth will eventually be lost anyway?

The source(s) of my fear or phobia is(are):

_____

_____

B. Degree of my fear or phobia

Am I fearful or phobic about dentistry?

1. *Fear Level One*

   • I visit the dentist on a regular basis, although I feel very apprehensive at each visit and I am very happy when the visit is over.
   • At my dental appointments, my heart pounds rapidly and my palms are sweaty. I may have other physical signs (Figure 1).

2. *Fear Level Two*

   • I don't visit the dentist unless I have an emergency or a toothache.

- I might go for a checkup once in a while, but not on a regular basis.
- I feel very apprehensive during each visit and can't wait till it's finished.

3. *Phobia Level One*

- I rarely visit a dentist and have not seen a dentist in many years.
- It is very hard for me to get numb — the novocaine never seems to work. I always have a lot of pain at the dental office.
- I know I have a lot of dental problems, but I just can't make myself go to the dentist.
- If I have a broken tooth, I would rather live with that than visit a dentist to have it repaired.
- Sometimes, I think I might pass out in the dentist's office.
- I have had dental emergencies that I have taken care of by myself.

4. *Phobia Level Two*

- I can identify with many of the statements in the preceding category.
- I feel depressed often.
- I feel life is going nowhere for me.
- Sometimes, I think I might die or kill someone in the dental office.
- I feel obsessed with a particular fear about dentistry.
- I really hate dentists.
- I feel that I may have other psychological problems.

My level of dental fear or phobia is: _____

My appropriate choice of treatment to overcome this fear is:

- ☐ selecting a gentle dentist.
- ☐ using the dental fear control program.
- ☐ having a support person help me to make an appointment.
- ☐ seeing a psychotherapist to help me feel more self-confident so I can deal with this fear or phobia.

3

THE PSYCHOLOGY AND PHYSIOLOGY OF DENTAL PAIN AND FEAR

Mary, an adult patient of mine for several years, had a generalized fear of dentistry stemming from bad childhood experiences. Despite this fear, she regularly kept her appointments for checkups every six months. Once she developed a toothache and needed treatment involving extensive drilling. The entire day before her appointment, she worried about what would happen during the drilling. She expected the worst. During her appointment, she did experience significant pain, as she had expected, and she required many shots of novocaine to dull the pain during drilling. Mary had programmed herself to feel pain. Figure 3 depicts a phobic's mental image of being tortured in the dental office. This situation is difficult for any dentist or any patient to deal with successfully.

Harriet, on the other hand, developed trust in me over the years and had confidence in her ability to remain calm in the dental chair. At her appointment for crown preparations (which involved lengthy drilling), she opted to have the procedure done without novocaine. During the two-

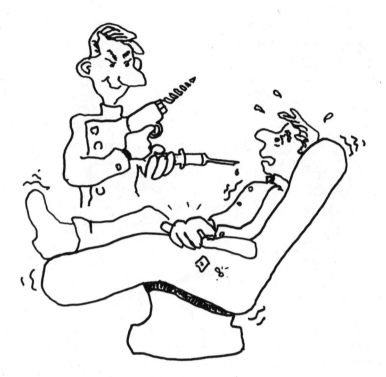

Phobic's mental image of dentistry

Fig. 3

hour procedure, she remained calm and had no apparent expressions of pain. When asked if she had any pain, she said that she felt only a minor amount of discomfort. Figure 4 gives an example of the relaxed patient's mental picture of dentistry.

Harriet and Mary are very similar persons: same sex, same socioeconomic background, same race, and the same age. They had similar procedures performed by the same dentist under identical conditions. However, their behaviors were strikingly different. While Mary required many novocaine injections, Harriet required none at all. Mary had significant pain and Harriet had only minor pain. Why?

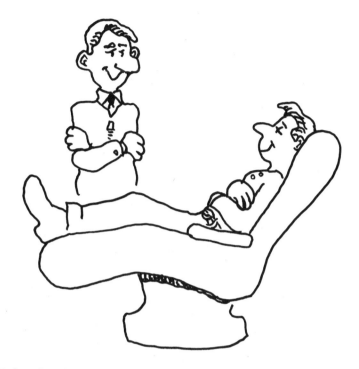

Relaxed patient's image of dentistry

Fig. 4

Mary and Harriet had different pain perception thresholds. They also had different psychological programming. Mary expected pain and Harriet did not.

In this chapter I will explain why people have different pain thresholds and why it is important to change your pain threshold so that you can tolerate dental procedures without repeated shots of novocaine. A person with a low pain threshold can raise it through a variety of methods. By understanding these concepts, you can gain better self-control and increase your self-confidence during your dental visits. This will not only help you but will also help your dentist perform the procedure more accurately.

Figure 5 shows the pathway of pain, which involves a rapid transmission of the pain impulse to the brain where it is interpreted as painful or as not painful. Three things can happen when pain is perceived: a reflex motor action (hand pulling away from fire), a psychosomatic reaction (nausea, heart beating rapidly, muscle tension), and storage of the painful experience in the memory bank of the brain.

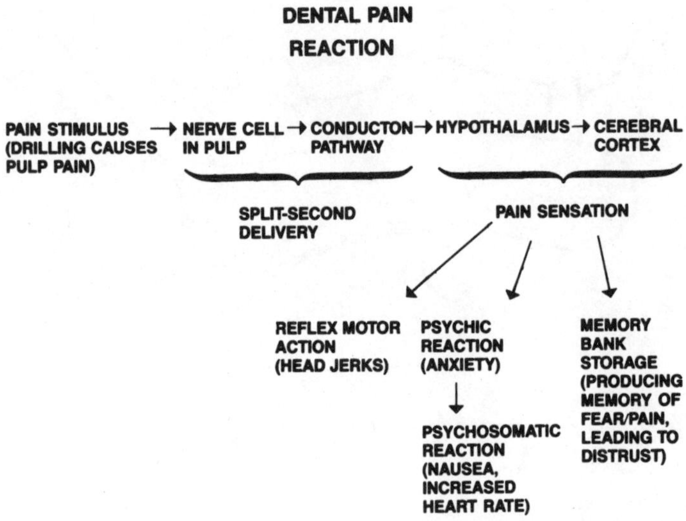

DENTAL PAIN REACTION

PAIN STIMULUS → NERVE CELL → CONDUCTON → HYPOTHALAMUS → CEREBRAL
(DRILLING CAUSES   IN PULP   PATHWAY   CORTEX
PULP PAIN)

SPLIT-SECOND   PAIN SENSATION
DELIVERY

REFLEX MOTOR   PSYCHIC   MEMORY
ACTION   REACTION   BANK
(HEAD JERKS)   (ANXIETY)   STORAGE
                              (PRODUCING
                              MEMORY OF
               PSYCHOSOMATIC FEAR/PAIN,
               REACTION   LEADING TO
               (NAUSEA,   DISTRUST)
               INCREASED
               HEART RATE)

From *Managing the Apprehensive Dental Patient.* Reprinted with permission.

Fig. 5

Fearful and painful episodes are stored in this memory bank. Research has shown that the memory bank is like a video recorder that can replay old memories with the original colors, sounds, sights, and, most significantly, the original emotions. Because past emotions are interwoven with painful past experiences, a person learns to associate a certain stimulus (the dental office) with the emotion of fear.

If the experience was particularly traumatic, fear may develop into a phobia.

For example, Kurt, a patient of mine, had dental phobia. He had been hurt in his childhood by a dentist who did not use any novocaine during drilling. As a college student, he had a toothache and visited a dentist who tried to extract the offending tooth. After some time the dentist found that he was unable to remove it. The dentist told Kurt to leave the office, even though by now he had more pain than when he first entered the office. With his tooth now traumatized from the attempted extraction, he was forced to seek help elsewhere. This was difficult because it was a Saturday afternoon. These events were recorded in Kurt's memory bank and helped to develop his dental phobia. When he finally came to my office for dental care, Kurt had many areas of decay in his mouth. He also had strong memories and a powerful phobic influence. In my office, Kurt received gentle care and he went through the dental fear control program (described in Chapter 5). He is currently having his mouth restored and he is gradually overcoming his dental phobia.

THE THREE PARTS OF PAIN

The three components of pain are physical, emotional, and evaluative. In their excellent book, *The Challenge of Pain*, Melzack and Wall give many examples of how these three components interact.

Physically, the pain impulse is carried to the brain by nerve fibers. Certain chemicals, bradykinin and histamine, are released at the site of the injury. These, together with other chemicals, can influence the severity of the pain impulse. Perhaps certain individuals have a genetic physical condition that allows them to feel more pain than others would feel under similar circumstances. However, I have seen very few (less than one percent) patients who do not respond well to a local anesthetic (such as novocaine) for pain control during dental treatment.

Emotions can significantly influence pain perception. High school football players emotionally involved in an intense game often ignore what would ordinarily be perceived as a painful injury. Dental patients, if under considerable stress (from the dental situation or in their personal life), may be more likely to experience pain during treatment. I have seen many, many fearful and phobic patients who, after they have learned effective relaxation exercises, do very well during their dental visits.

The *evaluative* component of pain involves self-talk, the thinking that occurs during an event. A person with negative self-talk, such as Mary (the first example in this chapter), will often experience more difficulty in a dental visit than someone who can think positive, happy thoughts. Examples of negative thoughts are: "This is awful — I think I'm going to die," "I know this is going to hurt (or I'm going to gag)," "I wonder when the pain will start and how bad it will be." Examples of positive self-talk are: "I know I can do this," "The dentist and his assistant are kind and gentle," "I know it's almost over," "I'm doing well and I feel good that I can do this." Positive thinking has been shown to produce great results for business executives and athletes. Dr. Denis Waitely, in his series *The Psychology of Winning*, has shown that successful people consistently think positive thoughts and always expect the best out of any situation. This attitude can be applied to the dental situation with predictably excellent results.

Pain is interpreted in the limbic system of the brain. This system regulates certain body functions such as blood flow. Through biofeedback, a person can learn how to regulate some of these functions which formerly were thought to be automatic. The reward and punishment center is also located in this section of the brain. This center is the basis for the behavioral school of psychology. Negative behavior (such as dental phobia) can be replaced with positive behav-

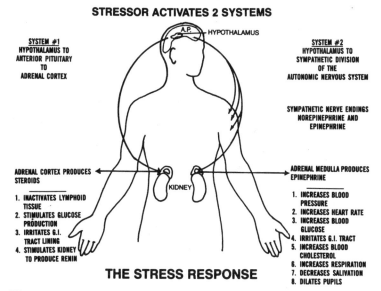

Fig. 6

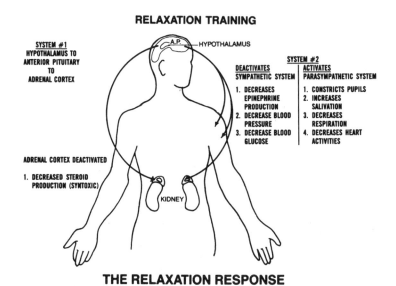

Fig. 7

ior (good dental visits). The psychosomatic center is also located here. This center can produce the stress or fear response (Figure 6) as well as the relaxation response. The stress response generally excites the body and, in the dental situation, can lead to an increased perception of pain. Likewise, the relaxation response (Figure 7) calms the body which can lead to a decreased perception of pain during dental treatment. It is impossible to be relaxed and tense at the same time. The body cannot generate both responses simultaneously. If a fearful patient can learn to produce the relaxation response naturally, chances are good that he or she will feel comfortable and have much less pain during treatment than someone who is fearful, tensed, and expects the worst.

THE GATE CONTROL THEORY

The gate control theory of pain correlates the psychological and physical factors of pain perception. The pain impulse generated in the receptor cell (such as drilling on a tooth) passes through the spinal cord to the brain (where it is then interpreted as painful or nonpainful). This area in the spinal cord is considered the "gate." This gate can open or close. As the pain impulse is sent from the gate to the brain, a signal is sent simultaneously from the brain to the gate. This signal, from a central control in the brain, can open or close the gate and thereby modify the pain impulse. If a person has had bad dental experiences which are now vividly stored in his or her memory bank and which make him or her afraid of the dental visit, and if this person expect the worst, then his or her control signals will tend to open the gate and allow the pain impulse to travel rapidly to the brain where he or she may experience significant pain. Figure 8 illustrates this concept. Thus a fearful patient may need extra shots of novocaine for adequate pain control.

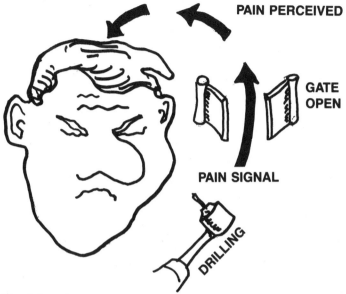

Fearful patient + gate open = more pain
Fig. 8

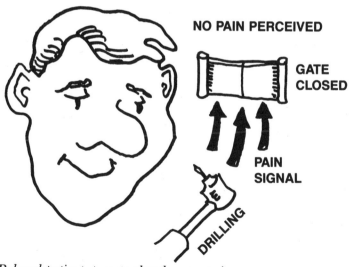

Relaxed patient + gate closed = no pain
Fig. 9

But if a patient has learned effective relaxation methods, if he or she has confidence in the dentist and staff, and if he uses positive self-talk, he may activate his control center to close the gate, thereby allowing the novocaine to be effective and reducing the chance of pain. Figure 9 illustrates this patient.

In understanding the gate control theory, there are three factors to consider: the sensation threshold of pain, the pain perception threshold, and pain tolerance.

Evidence shows that all people have a *uniform sensation threshold of pain.* If a group of people were pricked with a pin at the same time, they would feel the sensation of the pin prick simultaneously. However, their *pain perception thresholds* would be different, as would their abilities to endure continued pin pricks *(pain tolerance).* Why do people have different pain perception thresholds? Many factors determine a person's pain perception threshold and pain tolerance:

- cultural background
- early life experiences
- ethnic influences
- painful memories
- stress or fear level
- fear of not being able to control the situation
- negative self-talk

Since these are mainly learned experiences, behavior modification can help a person change his or her behavior to become relaxed in the dentist's chair.

Certain things can be done by the dentist and staff to help raise the pain perception threshold of the patient:

- relaxed office environment, including the overall design
- stereo headphones
- caring and friendly attitude of dentist and staff

- the dental fear control program
- effective local anesthetics
- pharmacological aids, if needed: nitrous oxide, pre-medication, or intravenous sedation
- listening, noncritical dialogue

Certain things can be done by the patient to achieve the same result:

- learning effective relaxation methods
- taking responsibility for one's level of fear/emotions
- positive self-talk
- developing trust in the dentist and staff
- learning distraction techniques
- becoming assertive in the dental chair (if it hurts, say something to the dentist)
- learning to feel a sense of control during dental treatment

Although a person might possibly be affected by a genetic factor predisposing him or her to an increased pain perception threshold, most dental phobics are influenced by negative behavior factors that can be unlearned.

The dentist and staff can do only so much. They must perform well (as described in Chapter 13) but they cannot be expected to produce perfect pain control for a highly charged, phobic individual who is unwilling to assume any responsibility for his or her fear level. However, in my experience, most patients perform extraordinarily well after learning effective behavioral methods, including relaxation exercises, that will be described in Chapter 4. Before learning these exercises, you should first understand sources of dental fear and dental phobia and where yours may have originated.

SELF-ASSESSMENT

1. How do I rate myself: fearful or phobic about dentistry?

   _____

   _____

   _____

   _____

2. Describe the three components of pain:

   - _____
   - _____
   - _____

3. Describe the gate control theory of pain and how it can affect me in the dental chair:

   _____

   _____

   _____

   _____

   _____

4. List some things I can do to raise my own pain perception level and become more comfortable in the dental chair:

   - _____
   - _____
   - _____
   - _____
   - _____

4

RELAXATION EXERCISES:
HOW THEY CAN WORK FOR YOU

Certain relaxation techniques can help the fearful patient successfully cope with the dental visit. These exercises can be used in the treatment room by both dentist and patient to make their interaction less stressful.

Four of these relaxation methods are paced breathing, meditation, progressive muscle relaxation, and guided imagery. By practicing the scripts that follow, you can learn the skills of progressive muscle relaxation and guided imagery and incorporate them into your daily life. These techniques can have a powerful relaxing effect on your body. Like anything else, the more you practice the skills, the more proficient you will become at relaxing yourself. If you are taking any medication, you should consult your physician for advice on dosage. Relaxation exercises work together with tranquilizers and certain other medicines to produce very deep relaxation. Dr. Herbert Benson, a Harvard University professor and author of the book, *The Relaxation Response,* demonstrates that his patients who have high blood pressure can permanently lower their blood pressure without medication by learning the relaxation skill of meditation.

The reason these relaxation exercises work is that it is impossible for the body to be tense and relaxed at the same time. The body is controlled by two nervous systems: a relaxation system and a tension system. When you initiate the relaxation system (whether you use a relaxation exercise or a tranquilizer), you automatically cancel out the stressful effect of the tension system. The two systems do not work together at the same time. If you can learn to produce relaxation, you can automatically cancel out the negative effects of the fear response.

Some fearful patients do not want to share any responsibility in reducing their fear level. They demand to be put to sleep for their dental treatment. Unfortunately, after having had their dentistry done under a general anesthetic, their fear remains and they continue to avoid dentists. Years later, their mouths have deteriorated again. So, in order to have a good long-term relationship with dentistry, the patient *must assume responsibility* for his or her fear. A major part of this responsibility is learning to relax in the dental chair.

Learning these exercises may take time. And nobody has time for things they really don't want to do. These exercises are effective in producing as much relaxation as a tranquilizer or nitrous oxide. The more you practice the exercise and the more you really believe in it, the more it will work for you.

PACED BREATHING

A useful, easy-to-learn relaxation method, is paced breathing or paced respiration. This technique has been used in the Orient for centuries. Although there are several variations of paced breathing, the basic idea is to slow down and regulate breathing in a uniform pattern.

Some fearful patients breathe rapidly and others hold their breath. These two extremes of breathing increase the stress response inside the body, causing the patient to actually become more anxious. To learn this relaxation method, begin by taking a deep breath for the count of five. Then hold the breath for five seconds. Then slowly exhale to the count of five. Breathing like this for 10 minutes will induce relaxation. The patient can easily perform this exercise while in the dentist's chair.

MEDITATION

Dr. Herbert Benson, in his laboratory at Harvard Medical School, has given scientific credibility to meditation as a useful tool in the healing arts. Dr. Benson has monitored the physiological responses and brain wave patterns of patients who become deeply relaxed using meditation alone. He found the following in patients who relaxed with meditation: decreased oxygen consumption, decreased respiratory rate, decreased heart rate, decreased blood pressure, decreased muscle tension, and increased alpha brain waves.

To be effective, meditation requires: a quiet environment, a comfortable and relaxed body posture, a passive attitude (to ignore distracting thoughts), and an object to dwell upon (called a mantra). A quiet environment is necessary because any disturbance can destroy the effect of relaxation. A passive attitude assures that you will not worry how well you are doing or if distracting thoughts occur. This nonchalant attitude is the frame of mind that is necessary for successful meditation and is perhaps the most important requirement for it.

To practice meditation (as described by Benson), put yourself in a comfortable position, loosen any tight clothing, and do everything possible to avoid interruptions. Relax yourself for ten minutes, using progressive muscle relaxation or paced respiration. Then, after this initial relaxation period, begin to repeat over and over again a mantra, such as the word, "Calm," or "Peace," or "Slow." If your mind wanders, return immediately to the mantra, although don't worry if such thoughts occur. Maintain a passive attitude throughout the entire meditation.

With practice, meditation can produce deep levels of relaxation. You can use this technique to relax before your dental visit, although you may have trouble using it during your visit because of the noise factor in a dental office.

PROGRESSIVE MUSCLE RELAXATION

Progressive muscle relaxation, first described by Dr. Edmund Jacobson in 1938, has been used by psychologists and psychiatrists extensively over the years. This technique reduces muscle tension (a symptom of fear) by progressively tensing and then relaxing all the major muscle groups of the body. It is easy to learn and does not require as much mental concentration as other techniques. However, it requires about 15 to 30 minutes for a profoundly relaxed state which is more time compared to the other methods. When combined with a mental technique, such as guided imagery, it becomes powerful. It is very useful for an apprehensive patient prior to an injection to decrease over-all muscle stiffness.

The following is a script from an audiocassette tape that I use in my office to teach relaxation to dental phobics and to patients under considerable stress with TMJ (temporomandibular joint) problems. On the first side of this tape is progressive muscle relaxation and on the reverse is guided imagery. You may purchase this tape by writing to: Heritage Communications, 11469 Lippelman Rd., Cincinnati, Ohio 45246.

You may also decide to make your own tape. If you do, remember to speak slowly with a calm voice. You might also consult your dentist to find a source for a relaxation tape. Some bookstores also carry similar tapes.

Now, as you read this script, sit back in a comfortable chair and loosen any tight clothing.

TAPE SCRIPT:
PROGRESSIVE MUSCLE RELAXATION

"This tape program has been designed to help you produce the relaxation response inside yourself, naturally, and without drugs. This relaxation response is so powerful that it will nullify any fearful or stressful response being produced by your body's hormones. You see, it is virtually impossible to be relaxed and tense at the same time. Your body will respond to your command to relax, if you can train it to do so. If you cannot learn relaxation skills, then your body, when confronted by a fearful or stressful situation, will automatically produce the fear response characterized by sweaty palms, a pounding heart, and rapid breathing. On the other hand, if you become proficient at producing the relaxation response, not only will you feel more at ease during your dental visit, but your body will be more receptive to the local anesthetic and the novocaine will actually work much better for you.

"Also, these important skills will help you not only to conquer the fear and stress of dental procedures, but also to deal with the stressful situations we *all* encounter in everyday life. If you are having problems with TMJ pain or if you have a habit of clenching or grinding your teeth, then learning these skills can help you.

"Learning these relaxation skills will take time and practice. As a child, you didn't learn to ride a bicycle overnight. Likewise, learning to produce the relaxation response through progressive muscle relaxation or imagery will take practice on your part. Lots of it. I would suggest that you practice with this tape twice a day. Find a place that is quiet, away from the dogs and the children, and practice. After a few weeks of daily practice, you should be an expert with these techniques.

"There are *millions* of persons just like yourself. Several studies have shown that many Americans *do not* visit a dentist because they have a crippling fear of dentistry. There are a lot of people just like you —scared to death of the dentist. Many people who do visit a dentist on a regular basis for a dental checkup are *still reluctant* and somewhat fearful about their visits. You may be surprised to know that there are many things that can be done for the patient who has fear of dentistry.

"The goal of this program is to help you overcome your fear of dentistry. It is not a *simple* task. You will have to spend *much time* and effort to overcome your fear. However, you will have a *great reward* - a much better feeling about yourself and a much healthier mouth *and* body! Take it one step at a time.

"Now, close your eyes, sit back, and relax. We will now begin to learn the skill of progressive muscle relaxation. You will not learn this in one sitting. It may take you several times before you begin to feel totally relaxed. After you have mastered this skill, you can use it about one or two hours before your dental appointment for additional relaxation. Again, when you practice at home, find a quiet place with no distractions, pets, or children. Also, sit in a comfortable chair. A hard, rigid chair is not conducive to the progressive relaxation of your muscles. Loosen any tight clothing, such as a belt or tie. Now, close your eyes and become very comfortable in the chair. Take a deep breath. Take a very deep breath. Hold the air inside yourself. Feel your chest muscles become tight and rigid. Hold the breath. Now slowly and evenly exhale and think of the word *calm*. Feel the relaxation in your chest as you slowly exhale. Feel the total relaxation in your chest muscles.

"Take another deep breath and hold it . . . Hold it some more . . . Now, slowly exhale and feel the air slowly escape through your mouth.

"Again, take another deep breath and hold it . . . Hold it some more . . . Feel the tension in your chest muscles. Now slowly exhale and feel the air slowly escape. Feel the chest muscles relaxing . . .

"Feel the warmth of relaxation coming upon you. Wait for a few moments and feel the relaxation . . .

"Now, relax the facial muscles and the muscles of the neck and shoulder areas. Begin to wrinkle your forehead. Wrinkle it as *firmly* as your can. Hold it . . . Feel the tension in your forehead muscle. Now, relax your forehead and feel the muscle relaxing. Feel the relaxation in your forehead.

"Now, wrinkle your forehead again. Hold the tension. Feel the tension. Hold it some more. Now relax. Feel the tension leaving and the good feeling of relaxation.

"Now, close your eyes as *hard* as you can. Tense your eyes as tightly as you can. Now hold it . . . hold it . . . now relax . . . Feel the relaxation . . . Now again close your eyes tightly and feel the tension. Hold it . . . Now relax and feel the tension leaving.

"Now, smile as widely as you can. Show all of your teeth. Stretch your lips as hard and as far apart as you can. Hold it . . . Feel the tension in your facial muscles. Now relax your face. Let your mouth relax. Feel the muscles slowly relax. Feel the warmth.

"Smile again as widely as you can. Hold it very wide . . . Hold it . . . Now relax. Feel the relaxation coming into your face . . . Total body relaxation . . . Calmness . . . Complete calmness.

"Now, clench your teeth together as hard as you can . . . Hold it . . . Now relax your mouth and let your jaws separate. Feel the muscles relaxing. Feel the tingling sensation . . . Calmness . . . Feel how good your muscles feel when they are relaxed.

"Push your tongue up into the roof of your mouth and feel the tension. Feel the tongue pushing hard against the roof of the mouth . . . Hold it . . . Now relax your tongue. Feel the relaxation . . . Calmness.

"Now squeeze your shoulders up to your neck as hard as you can . . . Hold it . . . Feel the tension in your shoulders and neck . . . Hold it . . . Now relax and let your shoulder *effortlessly* drop. Take a deep breath and exhale slowly . . . Feel the calm sensation coming everywhere throughout your body . . . (Pause 10 to 20 seconds.)

"Again, squeeze your shoulders towards your neck tightly. Feel the tension . . . Hold it . . . Hold it . . . Now relax and let your shoulders drop. Take a deep breath and relax . . . Feel your body relaxing.

"Now, tilt your head backwards as far as you can and feel the tension in your neck . . . Hold it . . . Hold it . . . Now relax and let your head drop forward . . . Feel the calm sensation.

"Tilt your head backwards again and hold it tightly . . . Feel the tension . . . Hold it . . . Hold it . . . Now relax and let your head effortlessly drop forward. Feel the muscles relax.

"Now, squeeze your shoulders and pull your shoulders straight backwards as far as you can. Feel the tension in your shoulders and chest . . . Hold it . . . Hold it . . . Now relax and let your shoulders drop forward. Feel the absence of tension. Feel the muscles relax. Take a deep breath and hold it. Hold it . . . Now gently exhale and feel total relaxation. Reflect for a moment with your head effortlessly bent forward, on the total relaxation coming into your body . . . (Pause here for a few seconds.) Feel the warmth . . . Feel the *calmness.*

"Now stretch your right arm out to your side and hold it there. Make a fist and tighten your right fist as hard as you can. Make it tighter . . . Hold it . . . Feel the tension in your fist and arm . . . Hold it . . . Now relax and let your arm drop to your side . . . Feel the complete relaxation.

"Now, repeat this with your left arm. Stretch your left arm out to your side and hold it there. Make a fist and tighten your left fist as tightly as you can. Hold it firmly . . . Hold it . . . Feel the tension . . . Now relax and let your arm drop to your side . . . Feel the warmth . . . Feel both your arms dropped at your side feeling very warm . . . very relaxed . . . very heavy . . . calmness.

"Concentrate on the relaxed sensation in your arms. Feel the calm coming over you. Take a deep breath . . . Hold it . . . Feel the tension in the chest . . . Now tighten your stomach as if you are trying to *protect* yourself from someone about to *punch* your *stomach*. Feel the stomach muscles tighten. Feel the skin become rigid. Now relax and feel the muscle tension leave your stomach. Feel the warmth . . . think of the word *calm* . . .

"Now, lift your right leg off the floor and stretch it out in front of you. Stretch your leg straight ahead as far as you can and feel the muscles in the leg becoming tight and rigid . . . Hold it . . . Hold it . . . Now let it drop to the floor and feel the heaviness and relaxation coming into your right leg . . . Keep your eyes closed and feel the heaviness in your right leg . . . Feel the warmth . . .

"Let us now repeat the procedure for the left leg. Stretch your left leg straight ahead and feel the muscles in your leg becoming tense and rigid . . . Hold it . . . Hold the tension in your leg . . . Now let your leg relax and drop to the floor. Feel the heaviness and relaxation in your leg . . . Calm . . . Warmth. Stretch your right leg forward again and this time extend your toes downward and away from you. You will feel tenseness in the arch of your foot and in the muscles of the lower and upper parts of your right leg. Hold it . . . Hold the tenseness . . . Hold it . . . Now let your leg drop and relax . . . Feel the warm relaxation . . .

"Now, let's repeat this exercise for the left leg. Stretch your left leg forward and extend your toes downward and away from you. You will feel tenseness in your foot and leg muscles. Hold the tension . . . Feel the rigid muscles . . . Hold it . . . Now let your leg drop and relax . . . Feel the tingling sensation and relaxation . . .

"Now, sit back and relax. Let your head drop forward *effortlessly*. Take a deep breath . . . Hold it . . . Hold it . . .

Now slowly exhale and smile. Feel the warm relaxation running throughout your body. Feel your facial muscles *relaxed*. Feel the relaxation in your *shoulder* and your neck. Feel the warm relaxed sensation tingling throughout your arms, your chest, your face and head, your legs . . .

"Now listen to the soft music and let your body totally relax . . . Feel the warmth . . . Feel the soft, gentle relaxation coming over you."

GUIDED IMAGERY

Imagery is a technique to train your mind to think about a pleasant thought. On the cassette tape I provide my phobic patients, progressive muscle relaxation is on the first side and guided imagery on the reverse. This allows the patient first to practice a fairly simple technique and, then, while relaxed, to graduate to a more sophisticated one. Some patients, after experimenting with both techniques, prefer one technique over the other. Others derive relaxation equally well from either method.

In this tape script, there are four scenes: the ocean beach, a deep green forest, the sky, and a harbor at sunset. As I explain to my patients, they may prefer one scene over another, and, if they have fears associated with any scene (such as fear of the water), to concentrate on another scene. So again, sit back, get comfortable and put yourself on a beautiful beach down in the warm Caribbean. (This can be even more valuable if you are reading this in a northern climate in the dead of winter.) These techniques are also excellent for management of the dental phobic from the standpoint of distraction in that they distract his attention away from the dental procedure.

TAPE SCRIPT: GUIDED IMAGERY

"This tape program has been designed to help you to produce the relaxation response. The objective of this side is to help you learn to relax yourself through imagery, which is the skill of creating a scene in your imagination. Relaxation guided imagery is the skill that will allow you to create a very calm scene in your mind. Your mind is a very powerful force. If you can learn to tap into this power, you can train your mind to produce wonderful, soothing relaxation all throughout your body. This complete relaxation can be so powerful that it can lower your blood pressure and give you a wonderful feeling of euphoria. Scientists estimate that we use only a fraction of the power of the mind. So if you can learn to tap into this powerful force, you will be pleasantly surprised that your dental visits will be so much easier for you.

"You can use this skill to relax yourself prior to your dental appointment or during the actual dental procedure in the treatment room. You can also use it during any other *stressful* situation that may occur in your life. Again, like the skill of progressive muscle relaxation, this skill will require daily practice to achieve good results.

"During this tape, you will imagine four scenes. First, sitting on a beach at the ocean; second, looking up at the sky on a warm summer's day; third, a deep, green forest; and fourth, a quiet harbor at sunset. During each of these, use your imagination to create the sounds, smells, and colors of the scene. After several *practice* sessions, you may decide that you can achieve the greatest amount of relaxation through one *particular* scene. During these scenes, you can use your muscle relaxation *skill* to add to your relaxation. Use whichever muscle group seems to work the *best* for you. We will give you suggestions, but feel free to use your favorite muscle. If any *other* thought enters your mind, push it out. Concentrate on the scene.

SCENE I - The Ocean

"Now, we will introduce the *first* scene. Take a deep breath and hold it . . . Hold it . . . Now slowly relase it and feel the air slowly escape . . . Feel the calm . . . Take a deep breath again . . . Hold it . . . Feel the tension . . . Hold it . . . Now release . . . *Total* release . . .

"You are sitting on a sandy beach. All alone on the beach. The waves are gently rolling up on the beach. The water is crystal clear and further down the beach, you can see a clear, blue color in the sea. The warm sea wind blows in on your face. Feel the warmth of the sea breeze. Take a deep breath. Feel the warm sand you are sitting on. Watch the waves of crystal clear water gently splash up on the beach. Feel the *salty* spray. Taste the *salt* in the air. Feel the warm golden rays of the sun on your face and shoulders. You are at peace. You are calm. Hear the gentle rumble of the waves. As you gaze out over the ocean, you can see a fishing boat, white with red trim, slowly making its way over the water. The day has been a good one for the fishermen and their nets are full of fish. As you watch the boat sail away into the horizon, becoming smaller and smaller, you can feel yourself becoming more and more relaxed.

"You now decide you're going to take a walk along the beach. As you walk toward the water's edge, you can feel your feet sink into the warm sand. As you wade into the water, you can feel the water splashing up onto your legs. The temperature of the water is warm and feels very comfortable to your skin. Your skin has slowly become very warm and relaxed.

"As you wade through the water, you notice the water is so crystal clear that you can see all the way to the ocean floor. And as you gaze down through the silver-blue water, you see a starfish on the ocean floor. A beautiful large starfish with five golden yellow arms radiating out from its body. A star of the sea.

"Up ahead, a school of tiny greenish blue fish glides by in formation, with the sunlight shooting a prism of colors as the fish change directions underwater. White sunshine flickers in the water's moving lens and reflects the whole scene.

"Further along the beach, you discover a sea shell. A large conch shell with a pearly pink mouth. The lining of shell's orifice is smooth and shiny, once a home for another sea creature. The shell's mottled surface, rust-colored and gnarled has been bleached and weathered by the wind, sun, and waves. As you hold the shell up to your ear, you can hear the faint sounds of the ocean, and the waves gently tumbling onto the beach.

SCENE II - The Sky

"Now, while still sitting at the beach, let us focus our attention on the wonderful blue sky overhead. Imagine the soft blue color of the sky. Lazy white clouds in a sapphire sea of blue. Take a deep breath and release it. Observe how relaxed you feel now, gazing up at the warm, blue sky. Feel the air and feel how fresh and relaxing it feels to look up at the sky on a warm summer day. How many colors of blue can you imagine in the sky? Some light blue, some dark blue, some turquoise, some aquamarine. See the soft rays of light beaming through the puffy white clouds, filtering down towards you. Feel the warm sunlight on your face. Take a deep breath and hold it. Feel the tension in your chest. Now release the breath and relax.

"What a wonderful day it is today! How good you feel — as if your entire body is radiating happiness! As you sit here, relaxed, gazing up at the sky, you can feel a warm breeze blowing across your face and shoulders. How good and warm that breeze makes your body feel.

"As you look up at the sky, you notice a sea gull circling around and over the water. As you watch the sea gull you notice the arc in his wings and the graceful movement of his body. His feathers glowing with brilliance, his wingtips moving in unison. Suddenly, the gull folds his wings and, for a moment, stands still in the sky, then begins a dive to the ocean, searching for food. Making a small splash in the water, the seagull now rises again, carried upwards by the powerful strokes of his wings. Rising up among the sun's rays filtering down, the gull forms a striking silhouette against the white banks of clouds. And, as the gull circles and glides, effortlessly, through the summer's sky, your thoughts turn to how relaxed you have become.

SCENE III - The Forest

"Now, let's switch scenes and move to the middle of a green forest. You are sitting down, looking out into an emerald sea of green leaves and tall trees. It is a cool, crisp morning. Sense the quiet of morning. There is some misty fog filtering through the forest. It gives an enchanting quality to the woods. The floor of the forest is covered with a carpet of green moss. Deep green ferns and other vegetation abound everywhere. Now, take a deep breath and hold it . . . Now release the air and feel the relaxation . . . Look up at the tall redwood trees. See how they tower up into the sky. Look at the massive strength in the trunks of the redwoods. Feel the freshness and quiet of the forest. Feel the stillness . . . In the middle of the forest, a quiet stream flows over a creekbed of rocks and stones. The water in the creek is sparkling and clear. It surges ahead with a feeling of freshness and clarity.

"Across from you, a squirrel dances along the forest's floor and hops up on a hollow log. Dwarfed by the giant redwoods, the squirrel grabs a nut and holds it like a prize. Sitting up on his hind legs, perched on the log, he is staring at you and watching your every movement, almost ready to start a conversation. Then, as quickly as he entered your privacy, he scampers away into the green haze of the forest.

"Next on the scene are two pesky chipmunks. Chitter-chattering between themselves, they run back and forth along the log, seemingly oblivious of you sitting among the tall redwoods. Their colorful, striped bodies seem to reflect their cheerful and playful personalities. Not a care in the world today, they hop and jump among the wildflowers. And, then, like the squirrel, they disappear into the forest.

"And, as you reflect on the beauty and peacefulness of this miniature ecology, you again feel deep and comfortable relaxation throughout your body.

SCENE IV - Sunset In The Harbor

"Now, let us switch to the final scene on the tape. Imagine yourself sitting on a dock at a harbor. It is sunset. The sun has drifted down beyond the clouds and boats and is casting an orange glow everywhere. A warm, orange glow. The sailboats lie quietly on the water, their solitary masts pointing upward. An aura of peacefulness and quiet penetrates the whole scene. The sunset paints everything orange — the water, the clouds, the entire sky. See the shadows of the sailboats reflected over the tiny ripples in the water. Feel the warmth of the orange sunset. Now take a deep breath and hold it . . . Feel the tension and release . . . Feel the ocean breeze blow in and smell the salt in the air. Feel the mystery and quiet of the sea.

"Listen, with your imagination, to the sounds of the waves rolling into the harbor. Listen as the waves lap up against the hulls of the boats. Hear the creaking of the masts and the sounds coming from the bellies of the boats.

"As you sit here, watching and feeling the perfect tranquility of the entire harbor, you notice the shifting of the clouds has created a rhapsody of color on the horizon. Purples blend into orange and oranges blend into reds and yellows. A cloud has exploded into a cauliflower-shaped mass colored in orange and purple. The brilliant purplish orange hue reflects over the shimmering ripples, painting the water with its colors, like an artist choosing from his palette of oils. As evening creeps in, the colors change to a blended combination of reds and purples.

"And, as you sit here, let your imagination paint this vivid scene of beauty and quiet stillness among the boats. Reflect, for a moment, on how relaxed you feel now, and listen to the soft sounds of the ocean."

Like anything else, these two skills require training and practice. The more you practice, the more skillful you become in producing the relaxation response. You may have attained some degree of relaxation by reading these two passages, but with practice, you will find it easier to become deeply relaxed.

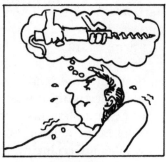 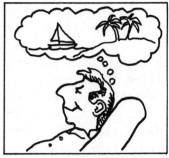

Tension   *Guided Imagery*

Your choice: tension or relaxation. Which will it be?

SELF-ASSESSMENT

Now that I understand that I can *deeply* relax myself with these natural relaxation exercises, I will try to commit myself to learning them through daily practice.

Commitments:

☐ I will make my own tape or have a friend help me.
☐ I will ask my dentist for a source of such a tape.
☐ I will order the tape through this publisher.
☐ I will practice these exercises daily.
☐ I will keep a daily log, recording hours practiced and noting my daily improvement.

Other goals:

_____

_____

_____

DAILY LOG FOR PRACTICE
OF RELAXATION EXERCISES

Day	Date	Time Spent	Results
Day 1	____	_____	_____
Day 2	____	_____	_____
Day 3	____	_____	_____
Day 4	____	_____	_____
Day 5	____	_____	_____
Day 6	____	_____	_____
Day 7	____	_____	_____
Day 8	____	_____	_____
Day 9	____	_____	_____
Day 10	____	_____	_____

Note: You can make copies of this log and tape it to your bathroom mirror where it will remind you to practice daily.

5

THE DENTAL
FEAR CONTROL PROGRAM

In the past, dental phobics have had their dental treatment performed under deep sedation, being either semi-conscious or completely asleep. While basic dentistry and oral surgery can be accomplished using general anesthesia, complex restorative procedures are difficult to accurately perform under these conditions. Also, the dental phobic remains in the grasp of the phobia, and usually will continue to avoid the dentist, resulting in oral deterioration.

In 1982, I developed a program to help dental phobics overcome their phobia naturally. In our office, the dental fear control program has helped more than 150 patients over the past five years. This system emphasizes patient responsibility in learning relaxation exercises and other methods to overcome fear. In a survey of these patients, 98 percent said that the program helped them overcome their fear and 70 percent said that they probably would not have returned for treatment if they had not gone through the fear control program.

In 1985, Dr. Timothy Smith, professor of psychology at

the University of Kentucky, organized a research project to develop a dental fear treatment network utilizing the dental fear control program. In the past two years, we have trained ten dental offices in Ohio, Kentucky, Indiana, and West Virginia. Data will be analyzed to determine the effectiveness of the program in these offices. Through additional seminars, we have trained other dental offices not associated with the research grant.

The net result is that I have seen many fearful and phobic patients tremble during their initial visit and then become calm after they had *taken the time* to go through the dental fear control program and learn relaxation exercises. They now have healthy mouths. They can smile again. Their self-images have improved dramatically. They also often tell me that they have advanced in their careers and have developed better social and family relationships.

Not all dental offices will have a formal program. Some offices use part of the dental fear control program and some dental fear clinics use similar behavioral programs. Your dentist may or may not use this program. However, by understanding these concepts and by practicing the exercises, *you* can accomplish much of the intended purpose of the program by *your own initiative.*

The program is divided into two sessions, usually one or two weeks apart. Some patients, feeling confident and relaxed after the first session, may not need to go through the second.

SESSION ONE

The first part of this session involves extensive interviewing to establish empathy and to determine the exact number(s) and severity of the dental fear(s). The patient completes several forms, the first of which is the dental fear self-analysis scale. Take a few minutes to complete this scale and try to be honest with yourself in rating your responses.

Although this scale is not scientifically proven, it may give you an idea of the relationship between the physical and psychological manifestations of dental fear. If you have a friend or relative nearby, you might discuss some of these questions with him or her. Add the numbers together so that you have a total score.

DENTAL FEAR SELF-ANALYSIS SCALE

Part I: Physical manifestations of dental fear

Close your eyes and let your imagination create this scene as vividly as possible. You walk into the dental office and the receptionist directs you to have a seat in the waiting room. Your appointment is for three fillings. You walk in and sit down. You fumble around for a cigarette to calm yourself down and notice the lack of ashtrays and the no smoking sign. You wonder whether the shot of novocaine is going to hurt. You wonder whether the dentist will hit a nerve during the drilling. How do you feel?

(circle one number per question)	Very much		So-so		Not at all
1. Do your palms feel sweaty?	5	4	3	2	1
2. Do you feel tense in general?	5	4	3	2	1
3. Does your stomach feel like it has butterflies?	5	4	3	2	1
4. Are you clenching your teeth now?	5	4	3	2	1
5. Does any muscle feel tight or tense anywhere in your body now?	5	4	3	2	1
6. Do you have a headache now?	5	4	3	2	1
7. Are you breathing heavily now?	5	4	3	2	1

The assistant greets you and asks you to follow her to the treatment room. She remarks on how nervous you look. The assistant seats you in the dental chair. You notice some of the dental instruments, which appear silvery and very sharp. One of them is curved like the horns of a bull. The dentist comes in and you lay your head back in the chair. He gives you an injection of novocaine and it feels as if the needle is going halfway down your throat. He waits a few minutes and then begins drilling on the tooth. You hear the high-pitched whine of the drill and it reminds you of a time long ago when a dentist hit a nerve while drilling on your tooth. The noise hurts your ears. Suddenly, you feel a sharp pain shooting from the tooth and traveling into your jaw-bone. Your head jerks involuntarily from the pain and the dentist looks at you and asks if that hurt you. You try to say something but your mouth is full of water, suction tips, a drill, and fingers. How do you feel now?

(circle one number per question)	Very much		So-so		Not at all
1. Do your palms feel sweaty?	5	4	3	2	1
2. Do you feel tense in general?	5	4	3	2	1
3. Does your stomach feel like it has butterflies?	5	4	3	2	1
4. Are you clenching your teeth now?	5	4	3	2	1
5. Does any muscle feel tight or tense anywhere in your body now?	5	4	3	2	1
6. Do you have a headache now?	5	4	3	2	1
7. Are you breathing heavily now?	5	4	3	2	1

Part II: The psychological aspects of dental fear.

(circle one number per question)	Terri-fied		So-so		Not afraid
1. How does the thought of a needle make you feel?	5	4	3	2	1
2. How does the thought of a needle in your mouth make you feel?	5	4	3	2	1

3. How does the thought of the
   drilling on one of your teeth make   5   4   3   2   1
   you feel?

4. Are you afraid you may be hurt
   during the drilling if the dentist   5   4   3   2   1
   should hit a nerve?

5. How does your image of dentistry   5   4   3   2   1
   make you feel?

6. How do the words "root canal,"
   "extraction," "oral surgery" make   5   4   3   2   1
   you feel?

Add up the total number of points and find your category below. If you did not feel many physical manifestations, try to imagine what you *actually* felt the last time you were in such a situation in the dental office. Be realistic.

100	Basket case
81 - 99	Petrified
61 - 80	Genuine fear
51 - 60	Frightened
41 - 50	Somewhat nervous
31 - 40	Mildly afraid
21 - 30	Cautious, but basically relaxed

Fear Analysis Scale Rating _____

The next form is a questionnaire to identify any fears you may have. Read this slowly and carefully and try to remember any events that may have caused you to develop any specific fear. Write down any bad experience(s) you may have had. Ideally you can discuss these fears with the dentist or his assistant so they know what really bothers you and so they can avoid causing the problem to recur. At the very least, you should be able to discuss these fears with a close friend or relative.

IDENTIFICATION OF YOUR DENTAL FEARS

1. As a child, did you ever have a bad dental experience? If yes, please write it down and describe it.

   _____

   _____

2. As an adult, did you ever have a bad dental experience? If yes, please describe.

   _____

   _____

3. Are you afraid of needles? If yes, please tell why.

   _____

   _____

4. Are you afraid of needles in your mouth?
5. Are you afraid of gagging? Please write down any bad experience.

   _____

   _____

6. Are you afraid the dentist will slip and cut your cheek?
7. Are you afraid you might do something that might be embarrassing to you in front of the dentist and the assistant?
8. Are you afraid you may be hurt during the drilling —if the dentist should hit a nerve? Please explain.

   _____

   _____

9. Does the sound of the drilling (high-pitched noise) bother you?

10. Are you afraid of the numbness produced by the injection?

11. Are you afraid you may choke during dental treatment?

12. Are you afraid of the unknown (not knowing what will happen once you are seated in the dentist's treatment room)?

13. Do you have fear of dentistry in general?

14. Were you ever physically assaulted around the face/mouth?

15. Do you have claustrophobia as applied to the dental office (fear of the dentist and assistant closing in or surrounding you)?

16. Do you have fear of invasion into the very private area of your mouth?

---

17. Do you have fear of rejection (if the dentist and assistant talk to each other and leave you out of the conversation)?

18. Do you have fear of fees (if they aren't explained to you ahead of time or if they surpass your budget)?

19. Do you have fear of an extraction?

---

20. Do you have fear of the smell of the dental office?

21. Do you have fear that the dentist will stick a sharp instrument (the "pick") into a sensitive part of your tooth?

22. Do you have fear of needing extensive dental treatment?

---

23. Do you have fear of the loss of your teeth?

24. Do you fear pain after the numbness has worn away?

25. Do you fear swelling after a procedure is done?

26. Do you have fear of any specific dental procedure —
teeth cleaning, root canal, crown, impressions, braces?

_____

27. Do you have fear of bleeding?
28. Do you fear that a disaster might happen in your
mouth?
29. Do you fear loss of control while you are reclined in the
dental chair during an appointment?

_____

30. Do you have any other fear or fears about dentistry?

_____

_____

This will initiate the process of catharsis, a cleansing
experience whereby a person unloads a painful or unhappy
memory. Imagine a person walking miles with a small pebble in his or her shoe. After the first mile, the pebble seems
like a boulder. Finally, after several miles, he removes the
pebble from his shoe and feels greatly relieved. So it is with
catharsis. A dental phobic with intense fears has avoided
dentistry for many years, his or her mouth deteriorating
year after year. Finally, he expresses his fears and overcomes
them, feeling like a new person again.

The next step is to watch a videotape showing the dentist
treating a fearful patient. Although this may not be available
to you, your dentist may allow you to watch him treating one
of his patients during an actual appointment. Your dentist
may have other videotapes that demonstrate some aspect of
dental treatment that may be worthwhile for your viewing.
In our videotape, I perform a routine dental filling on a
fearful patient. I demonstrate the following: a gentle injection of novocaine with a topical numbing cream, drilling
procedures, patient raising hand to stop the procedure,

stereo headphones to block out noise, nitrous oxide-oxygen conscious sedation, and the patient's reaction to the entire procedure.

Many dental phobics remember only the worst parts of their past dental experiences and their active imaginations balloon the situation way out of proportion. They report that watching the videotape helps them to see dentistry being performed in a modern setting with gentle techniques. They can identify with the fearful patient being treated. This helps them visualize themselves in his spot. However, some patients who are severely phobic cannot or do not want to watch this tape initially. They may need to wait until their confidence builds before watching it.

The next step in the program incorporates learning two relaxation methods: progressive muscle relaxation and guided imagery. These two methods were described in Chapter 4. In our office, we train our patients with the use of an audiocassette tape that contains instructions for these two techniques.

These relaxation exercises can be as effective as nitrous oxide or even intravenous sedation. I have seen patients fall asleep when using these methods. However, as with anything else, becoming skilled with these exercises requires practice. We advise our patients to practice with the tape for one or two hours each day for one to two weeks. At this initial session, the patient may decide to have his or her mouth examined or he may decide to have this done at a future appointment.

SESSION TWO

After you have practiced for one or two weeks with the relaxation tape, you should be well-versed in producing profound natural relaxation. If you have had trouble making time for this practice, refer to the end of this chapter for some ideas about this.

To begin this session, repeat the dental fear self-analysis scale to see what progress you have made. It will be helpful if you have also visited a dental office in conjunction with this first and second session, since your actual presence in the office will help to begin the deprogramming of your fear.

In our office, the next step is for the patient to practice a relaxation exercise (either one) for 10 to 15 minutes to become relaxed. Then, while relaxed, the patient watches the videotape again.

After watching the videotape, the patient begins a process called systematic desensitization, a scientifically proven method of reducing fear. Most experts agree that the basic therapeutic principle in overcoming fears and phobias is direct confrontation with the feared object or activity, ideally done without drugs. After the dental phobic faces the dental situation time and time again, his or her phobia gradually lessens and he becomes desensitized.

Before the patient is physically exposed to dental treatment, he or she can be mentally exposed to the fear-provoking stimuli by visualizing feared scenarios. This is done through systematic desensitization using guided imagery. The dental assistant or a friend or relative can read to you the following series of scenes. Then, while relaxed, you will gradually becomed desensitized. The scenes gradually increase in intensity. You can customize this "fear ladder" by adding any particular fears you may have at the end of the ladder. For example, if you have a fear of gagging, you might insert, after scene 8, a scene describing the dentist making an impression of your teeth. In this scene, you may imagine yourself feeling the urge to gag. Make this your customized fear ladder.

Systematic Desensitization

1. Use guided imagery or progressive muscle relaxation to achieve a relaxed state. Get into a comfortable chair

and loosen any tight clothing. Relax for about 10 minutes.
2. Read the scene. Visualize it. For example, imagine yourself calling to make a dental appointment.
3. After visualizing the scene for 10 to 15 seconds, use imagery or progressive muscle relaxation to calm yourself and remove the fear response. Use this relaxation for 30 seconds or more until the fear is gone.
4. Proceed to the next scene with this same technique.

DESENSITIZATION LADDER

1. *Calling to make an appointment.* You know it has been a long time since your last dental visit, and you remember the pain of a bad dental experience years ago. But your toothache is killing you and you know you must call. You pick up the phone and talk to the receptionist. She gives you an appointment.

   • Visualize this scene for 15 seconds. You may feel fear developing.
   • Use either relaxation exercise to remove your fear and produce relaxation. When the fear is gone, stop the relaxation process and proceed to the next scene.

2. *Driving to the dental office.* As you are driving to the office you again think back to your bad dental experience. You hope that it won't happen again today. You are not sure what's going to happen and you begin to wonder about the unknown.

   • Visualize this scene, relax, and repeat this process for the remainder of the scenes.

3. *Parking your car in the dental office lot.* As you pull your car into the lot, you begin to feel your palms sweat. You can feel the steering wheel becoming a little slippery from your sweat. You get out of your car and walk into the office.

4. *Entering the office.* As you walk through the door to the office, you can feel the fear building up and your heart beginning to pound. You tell the receptionist your name and you have a seat in the reception room. Your palms still feel sweaty.

5. *Entering the treatment room.* The dental assistant calls your name and escorts you into the treatment room. The dental assistant is friendly and tries to put you at ease. However, now, in addition to sweaty palms and a racing heart, your stomach feels like a bunch of butterflies.

6. *Dentist examines your tooth.* The dentist enters the room and introduces himself or herself and asks you if you are having a good day. Wonderful, you think. Your heart is beating so hard you think it will jump out of your chest. The dentist assures you he will be very gentle and that he has treated many fearful patients just like you. The dentist examines your tooth.

7. *An X ray is taken.* After examining your tooth, the dentist has decided an X ray is necessary for a complete diagnosis. You become very concerned about gagging. The assistant places a heavy lead shield around your body for protection and places the X-ray film in your mouth. It feels a bit uncomfortable, but you know it will be for only a few more seconds. The X ray is taken.

8. *The dentist explains the diagnosis.* The dentist sees the developed X ray and tells you the tooth has an abscess. However, he says it can be saved by removing the infected nerve. You are very happy the tooth can be saved and you are surprised that the dentist did not criticize you for having such badly decayed teeth.

9. *Dentist gives an injection.* The dentist asks you about having an injection and you tell him you are very afraid of needles. The dentist tells you he can be very gentle and to close your eyes if you desire. The dentist applies a topical cream to deaden the surface of the gums and then injects the needle into the gum. You feel a slight

sensation and then some pressure.

10. *Drilling begins.* The dentist has waited for the tooth to become profoundly numb. He then tells you he is about to start drilling and that if anything bothers you, raise your hand and he will stop immediately, because he does not want to cause you any pain. Your heart is pounding again and your stomach muscles feel very tight. The dentist drills on the tooth and soon you begin to smell a foul odor. He tells you this is gas escaping from the infected nerve in the tooth.

11. *You have pain during drilling.* During the drilling, you suddenly experience a sharp burning pain in your tooth and your hand shoots up. Sure enough, the dentist stops drilling as he promised and reinjects around the tooth. Soon he begins drilling again and finishes the treatment.

12. *You leave the office.* The procedure is finished. You are surprised at how gentle the dentist was and how caring and kind all the assistants were. You make an appointment for a complete checkup and leave happily. You are excited about telling your friends and relatives how nicely this office treated you and how well you did.

The principle behind desensitization is that it is physically impossible for a person to be relaxed and tense at the same time. By learning and practicing the methods in the dental fear control program, the fearful patient gradually raises his or her pain perception threshold. This helps the dentist and staff to complete treatment effectively. However, some people have trouble finding the time to practice these techniques. Several ideas may help you here to accomplish the goal of learning relaxation skills:

1. Find a quiet room, away from children, dogs, and so on.
2. Find a support person to help you each day.
3. Don't blame and berate yourself excessively for missing the practice sessions.

4. Look at your schedule. When can you find time? Set aside a specific time for practice each day.
5. Start a practice log and post this on your bathroom mirror where you will see it daily.
6. Evaluate any problems that cause you to miss practice.
7. Do the practice even if you don't feel like doing it.
8. Ask your support person or your dentist for helpful hints on practicing.

At the end of the second session, the patient is encouraged to continue practicing with the relaxation cassette tape and to also practice with the desensitization ladder on a daily basis. An appointment is then set for some type of dental treatment, if necessary.

For some people with excessive phobia or other fears besides dentistry, additional psychological treatment may be required. This can be done by a clinical psychologist or a psychiatrist, which will be described in the next chapter.

SELF-ASSESSMENT

1. What was my rating on the dental fear self-analysis scale?
   — initially _____
   — after 1-2 weeks of practice (with relaxation exercises) _____

2. If my dentist does not have a videotape of one of his or her procedures, will he allow me to watch him in action?
3. Do I have a log for my practice with relaxation exercises and systematic desensitization?
4. Who would be a good support person for me?

6

BIOFEEDBACK AND SELF-HYPNOSIS

We all march to the beat of different drummers. What might appeal to one individual may be repulsive to another. What might help one dental phobic relax might not help another. If progressive muscle relaxation or guided imagery are not as effective for you as you'd like, consider trying biofeedback or self-hypnosis. These techniques have been researched over the years and have been shown to produce deep states of relaxation.

BIOFEEDBACK

When fearful patients undergo dental treatment without any relaxation training, they experience many physical signs, such as rapid heartbeat, sweaty palms, rapid breathing, increased muscle tension, dry mouth, perspiration, and stomach butterfies or nausea. Becoming aware of these physical signs may lead you to feel more frightened than if those signs were not present.

Now, if you can learn to reverse these signs and change your "automatic" body response, will your fear decrease? This is the premise of biofeedback. You learn to regulate body functions, such as heartbeat and skin temperature, by directly observing feedback from your body. The biofeedback diagram (Figure 10) shows how this method works.

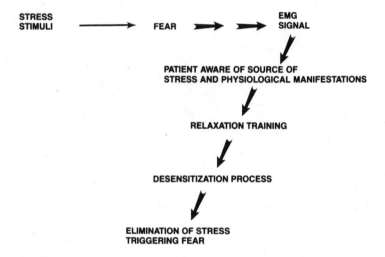

Biofeedback Diagram

Fig. 10

This technique may help those patients who feel that they have no control over their heartbeat during an injection or during dental treatment. Some of these patients feel that their body goes "haywire" when they get into the dental chair. Other patients who cannot readily detect their fear may benefit from biofeedback since they can see or hear an immediate replay from their body responding physiologically to the fearful stimulus.

In a research study to determine whether biofeedback could be helpful in decreasing dental fear, Dr. Richard Hirschman used an electromyographic (EMG) device to monitor muscle tension. This device (see Figure 11) measures electricity generated by muscle activity. Electrodes are placed on a specific muscle, and these run to a machine that delivers an audible or visual registration of muscle tension. The more muscle tension (as when a patient is highly fearful), the more electricity generated and the higher response on the EMG machine.

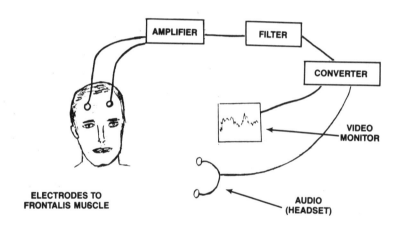

Biofeedback System

Fig. 11

Dr. Hirschman trained his patients to relax the muscle in the forearm while hooked up to the EMG machine. The patients noted that when they practiced relaxation, their arms became relaxed and the feedback was less intense. Dr. Hirschman found that fearful patients who received bio-

feedback training were less anxious during dental treatment than those who did not receive the training.

What body functions can a person regulate? Someone
who has had sufficient training in biofeedback can control
the following:

- Heart rate — the rate of blood flow as pumped by the
  heart.

It can be measured by a pulse meter, a simple device that
attaches to the finger and provides an electronic display of
the pulse. Some athletes wear a watch that displays the pulse
so that they can determine the degree of their training.

- Skin temperature, regulated by an over- or undersupply
  of blood (supplying warmth) near the surface of the skin.

In times of stress, a chemical message is relayed to the
skin's blood vessels, constricting them. This action pushes
the blood from the skin to the heart. Since the warmth
associated with blood is decreased in the skin, the skin
temperature falls in a stressful situation such as an injection
of novocaine. It can be measured by various devices that
attach sensors to the skin and feed this information back
either through audio or video means.

- Muscle tension — the amount of electrical energy in a
  muscle.

It can be measured by the electromyogram (EMG), a
device that can feed back audio or video signals indicating
the tenseness of a muscle.

- Galvanic skin response — the electrical resistance in the
  skin.

Changes in the electrical energy in the skin can be seen
on a monitor, in times of fear. The higher the frequency of
such changes, the more fearful the event. It can be measured by a galvanic skin response monitor that records

information in a manner similar to a lie detector (polygraph) machine.

An assortment of biofeedback devices measure these conditions:

- A pulse meter attaches to the finger with a digital display of the pulse. The higher the number, the higher the pulse (heart rate) and the higher the fear level. Cost is around $30.
- Skin temperature trainers are available in various devices at varying costs.
- A galvanic skin response monitor fits in the palm of the hand, allowing the fingers to rest on built-in sensing plates. This emits a tone that increases in pitch with fear and decreases with relaxation. Cost varies with the quality of the unit ($14 to $50).
- An electromyogram system feeds back signals based on the electrical activity in muscles. This signal can be heard or seen on a monitor. Many different devices are available, ranging in cost from $150 for a simple headset to thousands of dollars for a professional system.

These products are becoming readily available through stores such as Sears or Radio Shack. They are also sold through the following home shopping catalogs:

- New Horizons. Phone 1-800-453-9700
- The Sharper Image. Phone 1-800-227-3826
- Vital Concepts. Phone 1-800-642-8482

Please note that these catalogs may or may not offer these products at the time you read this book.

Another source of information on biofeedback is the Biofeedback Society of America, which also can supply a listing of dentists, physicians, and psychologists who practice biofeedback. The address is: Biofeedback Society of America, 4301 Owens St., Wheat Ridge, Colorado 80033.

HOW TO START BIOFEEDBACK

In order to benefit from biofeedback, you must be skilled in using a natural relaxation exercise such as the following (described in Chapter 4):

- Progressive muscle relaxation. This skill involves the alternate tensing and relaxing of all major muscle groups in the body.
- Guided imagery. Visualizing happy and tranquil scenes can be extremely effective in producing relaxation.
- Paced breathing. In this technique, you breathe at a much slower rate than normal. For example, when inhaling a breath of air, you count to five, hold the breath for five seconds, and then release over a period of five seconds. This technique has been shown to be effective in producing relaxation and is easy to do while in the dental chair.

PRACTICING BIOFEEDBACK

An effective way to reduce the fear response is by combining biofeedback with desenstization. You will need three things for this:

1. A mastered skill in a relaxation method such as progressive muscle relaxation, guided imagery, or slow breathing.
2. A biofeedback monitoring device. I would suggest a simple pulse meter.
3. A desensitization fear ladder. Arrange your fears about dentistry beginning with the least fearful scene and progressing to the most feared aspect of dentistry for you. For a sample fear ladder, you can refer to Chapter 5.

Step 1   Attach the pulse meter to your finger and take a reading while sitting in a comfortable position. Initial baseline pulse reading _____

Step 2   Look at your fear ladder and imagine the first scene. As you become apprehensive, you may note that your pulse rate increases. Record this in your log.

Pulse reading after first scene _____

Step 3   Now begin to practice your relaxation exercise to move your pulse back to the initial baseline pulse reading. Note how many minutes or seconds it takes you to do this.

Pulse reading after relaxation exercise _____

Time required to achieve this rate _____

It is a good idea to keep track of your practices in a log. In so doing, you can see your progress over a period of time.

PRACTICE LOG FOR
BIOFEEDBACK/DESENSITIZATION

Date _____   Time _____   Baseline pulse _____

	Pulse after scene	Pulse after relaxing	Time required
Scene 1	_____	_____	_____
Scene 2	_____	_____	_____
Scene 3	_____	_____	_____
Scene 4	_____	_____	_____
Scene 5	_____	_____	_____

You can make copies of this log for your daily practice and customize it according to your needs. With practice, you will feel a pride of accomplishment in noting your gradual improvement. This will reinforce your feelings of self-confidence in dealing with a dental situation. As your self-confidence builds, your fear will decrease. Gradually, you can apply this technique to the actual dental office environment.

SELF-HYPNOSIS

Hypnosis has been used over the last 200 years. Today, hypnosis is gaining more respectability in society. Several books ("Helping Yourself with Self-Hypnosis" by Caprio and "Self Hypnotism" by LeCron) have been written on this topic. Witnesses to crimes are sometimes put under hypnosis to elicit information. People take courses on hypnosis to lose weight or stop smoking.

However, several myths still surround hypnosis, keeping many individuals from using it:

Myth 1   "I cannot be hypnotized." It is estimated that only about 5 percent of normal adults cannot be hypnotized. Two important aspects of being hypnotized are a *deep desire to* be *hypnotized* and a *trusting relationship* with the person doing the hypnotizing (unless self-hypnosis is being used).

Myth 2   "I can be made to do something foolish while under hypnosis, possibly against my will." All hypnosis is essentially self-hypnosis. The person hypnotized does not lose control. In fact, the person hypnotized can learn to control such things as blood flow and other functions.

Myth 3   "I may not come out of the trance." Because the person being hypnotized controls himself, he can come out of the trance, if necessary.

Myth 4   "Hypnosis is the work of the devil." Totally unfounded. To the contrary, hypnosis has helped many thousands of individuals in many ways.

Hypnosis works only if you want it to work. Everyone has

the untapped potential that can be energized by hypnosis. If you really want to overcome your problem and be *in control* of your situation, you will benefit from hypnosis. The passive, dependent person who expects hypnosis to produce a miracle cure will usually be disappointed.

Many psychotherapists and other health professionals use hypnosis in their clinical practices. For a listing of such professionals, you can write to: American Society of Clinical Hypnosis, 2400 E. Devon Ave., Suite 218, Des Plaines, Ill. 60018.

Hypnosis is probably learned most effectively through a trained professional. However, some highly motivated people can learn self-hypnosis. Self-hypnosis consists of three phases: induction, trance or deep relaxation, and emergence.

1. *The induction phase.* You can use many methods to induce hypnosis. Two reliable methods are progressive muscle relaxation and guided imagery. If you become extremely proficient with these, you can arrive at a deep state of relaxation. This obviously takes much practice.
2. *The trance or state of deep relaxation.* In this phase, you are deeply relaxed. During the induction, suggestions may be given for you to become more and more deeply relaxed. In a state of deep relaxation, your subconscious mind becomes open to your programming. In this state, suggestions (such as those to decrease fear, appetite, and so on) may be programmed into the subconscious mind.
3. *The emergence phase.* Here, you emerge from deep relaxation. This normally happens when you decide you are ready.

A SAMPLE EXERCISE IN SELF-HYPNOSIS

1. Choose a quiet room without distractions or noise. This is important in achieving good results. Sit in a relaxed

position in a comfortable chair. Loosen any tight clothing.

2. Begin by making an audiocassette tape of guided imagery, progressive muscle relaxation, or some other method to achieve a deep state of relaxation. This tape could have 15 to 20 minutes of relaxation exercises followed by 5 to 10 minutes of suggestions for the subconscious mind. These suggestions would be customized for your own particular fears. The following may serve as a guide:

- I am becoming very skilled in producing deep relaxation.
- I want to save my teeth.
- I can control my dental fears.
- I can accomplish whatever I want to, if I put my mind to it.
- I can learn to trust my dentist and his or her staff.
- I'm getting better and better at visiting the dentist.
- I can relax in the dental office — I'm in control.
- I know the dentist will stop if I raise my hand.
- If I feel nervous, I can use my exercises to stop the fear.
- I can use my guided imagery to distract me during treatment.
- I can handle getting an injection of novocaine.
- I can handle the drilling. It won't last forever.
- The dentist is almost finished now.
- The dentist and his or her staff seem to be really caring about my fears. They take their time with me. I don't feel rushed.
- After my dental treatment is completed, I want to return on a regular basis for my preventive checkups. If I can overcome my fear, I can return for my checkups.

Use any positive statement that you think might help improve your attitude toward dentistry.

3. When the tape ends, you may stay relaxed and think over these thoughts. You may end the relaxation session whenever you choose.

You might consider doing this exercise in self-hypnosis before bedtime each night. You might also do it before each dental visit to reinforce your commitment to yourself and to your goals. It is interesting to note that when the subconscious mind is programmed with positive thoughts, you usually carry out those thoughts successfully.

The two additional relaxation strategies presented in this chapter may or may not help you. Some people need extra help: the special insight and training of a psychotherapist, which is the subject of the next chapter.

7

HOW PSYCHOTHERAPY CAN HELP

Do you need to seek professional counseling from a psychologist or a psychiatrist? This is a question that is, perhaps, not easy to answer. The majority of my fearful or phobic dental patients do well enough with the coping strategies described in this book and are able to have their dental treatment completed. However, occasionally a patient will not have complete success with these methods and will require psychotherapy. Consider some cases that I did refer for psychological help. By evaluating these patients, you may be able to decide whether you need to see a mental health professional.

Sally had a tremendous fear of gagging and said that she would often gag while eating. In dentistry, many procedures, ranging from simple X rays to fillings and impressions, can easily cause this type of person to gag. Initially, X rays were taken for Sally as part of her examination. During these X rays, Sally was uncomfortable and gagged. She tried many techniques to offset this tendency, but with limited success.

I explained to Sally that a friend of mine, a clinical psychologist, worked with patients who had trouble with gagging. She consented to see the psychologist. During her psychological treatment, Sally learned to use hypnosis to cope with her gagging problem. After a few sessions with the psychologist, Sally returned brimming with confidence. She told me that she no longer gagged while eating and felt much better now that she had learned to deal with this problem. I noticed that Sally was much more relaxed in the dental chair than previously. After the sessions with the psychologist, she had only minor problems with gagging and was able to have her treatment successfully completed.

Severe gagging can be a real problem for the dental patient. The source of gagging can be either physical and anatomical or psychological. Some people have difficulty wearing an upper denture because they gag when it is inserted. They have an unusual anatomy of the roof of the mouth. These people will be able to wear the denture if the rear part of it is trimmed far enough so that the gag reflex is not stimulated. This type of patient is usually not fearful.

If the gagging stems from a psychological basis, then psychotherapy can help. Hypnosis and nitrous oxide are effective in reducing gagging. These methods produce deep relaxation which may relax the muscles that cause the gag reflex. If a person is fearful and tense, his or her muscles tighten. This can explain the psychological basis of gagging.

A patient of mine for a few years, Joan was always somewhat apprehensive about dental treatment. She had complete confidence in me, however, which allowed her to feel relaxed enough to have her treatment performed. Initially, she decided she did not need the dental fear control program.

On vacation in Florida, she had an accident. Walking out of a restaurant, Joan tripped and fell face first into the sidewalk. Her lips were scraped, and her teeth were chipped and loosened by this severe blow. Unwilling to trust anyone else to treat her, she called me from Florida, described the accident, and told me she was going to drive nonstop to Cincinnati to see me. When she arrived, I noticed she was upset and shaken by this accident, but I was able to treat her dental emergencies successfully.

Over the next year, Joan began to cancel her appointments. When this became a regular pattern, I called her and asked about it. She told me she felt bad about canceling, but every time she had an appointment she developed many physical problems. She said she would begin to shake, and feel nauseated and light-headed. I told her that this was unusual and not normal. I said that it could be psychosomatic because it happened only when she prepared to visit the dentist. I suggested that she seek psychological help, since she might have another problem in addition to her dental phobia.

After a few weeks, she called me, explaining that she did consult with a psychologist, who diagnosed her problem as *panic attacks*. This condition causes a person to have an overwhelming feeling of impending doom characterized by pounding heart and other physical symptoms. People with these feelings often do not want to leave their home because they fear having a panic attack in public. This was Joan's problem. She was treated by the psychologist successfully and then returned to me for the remainder of her dental treatment. She was extremely grateful to me for suggesting that she seek professional counseling.

A third case was Elaine who was referred to my office by an oral surgeon she had consulted. Elaine had much dental disease, many decayed teeth, and advanced gum problems. She was a candidate for an overdenture, where a few roots of teeth are saved to anchor the dentures more securely than if no teeth were saved at all.

Elaine was holding a stuffed toy clown when she came to my office. She said that she had been through many medical procedures throughout her life and that she hated all doctors and dentists. She said she was extremely fearful of having anything done in her mouth. She mentioned, while in the treatment room, that she felt that she might die — or kill somebody. At this remark, my assistant decided to leave the room. She made other statements which seemed inconsistent or irrational. When I suggested that she go through our dental fear control program, she refused, stating that she had already tried these techniques and that her fear wasn't all that bad. When I questioned her about dental treatment, she again told me that she was terrified of it.

I became concerned during this initial interview, because I could not communicate well with her. When I asked her a question, she often would make a statement totally unrelated to the question. She wanted to dictate to me the exact treatment she wanted. However, some of her requests were technically impossible.

I wanted to try to save some of her remaining teeth as supports for an overdenture, so I referred her to a nearby periodontist (gum specialist), who would decide whether the teeth were salvageable. The periodontist thought that this patient would be extremely difficult to work with to save some teeth for the overdenture.

A referral to the Dental Fears Treatment Clinic at the University of Kentucky seemed to be in order. Elaine drove to Lexington, where Dr. Timothy Smith, a research psychologist at the university, was able to help her accept dental care. The staff at the clinic thought that all teeth should be removed and complete dentures made. This was done successfully. Dr. Smith describes this patient in the next chapter.

These three cases illustrate how patients can be helped by psychotherapy. Dentists are not trained to make a diagnosis of a psychological condition. Some patients do not respond well to conventional treatment, such as the dental fear control program, and require help elsewhere.

WHEN AND WHERE TO GET HELP

When should you think about consulting someone for psychotherapy? Ask yourself whether any of these statements apply to you:

- You have a deep desire to save your teeth.
- You feel you can't deal with having dental work done while you are awake.
- You don't want to be put to sleep for treatment.
- You like the dentist you're seeing at present.
- You feel as if you might have a panic attack at the dentist's office.
- You feel depressed often, especially about your teeth.

Where, then, should one seek help? Three sources of help are available: the psychologist, the psychiatrist, and the mental health center.

1. The clinical psychologist is licensed by the state to practice clinical psychology. He or she holds a doctoral degree (Ph.D. or equivalent) and can use a variety of methods to help you overcome dental fear. The psychologist cannot, however, prescribe medications, such as tranquilizers.
2. The psychiatrist is licensed by the state to practice medicine. He or she holds an M.D. degree and can use several methods to treat phobias, including the prescription of medications.
3. Mental health centers are dedicated to helping patients with a variety of psychological problems. The staff may be composed of psychologists, psychiatrists, or other professionals. If you live in a rural area that does not have a psychologist or a psychiatrist in private practice, you may be able to locate a mental health center.

When you decide to call for help, be sure to ask the

psychologist or psychiatrist whether he or she is interested in treating dental phobics. Does he have any experience with such patients? If you do not know who to call, ask your dentist, if you currently have one. You may also ask your physician for a referral. Other sources of referral for psychotherapy are:

1. Local academy of clinical psychologists. You may be able to find this listing in the yellow pages of your phone book.
2. Local academy of physicians. They would be able to give you the name of a psychiatrist who treats patients with phobias.
3. The Phobia Society of America. By writing or calling, you might be able to find a professional in your area who treats phobias. Address: 133 Rollins Ave. — Suite 4B, Rockville, Md. 20852. Phone: (301) 231-9350.
4. The Society of Behavioral Medicine. By writing, you might obtain a directory of psychologists to find one in your area. Address: P.O. Box 8530, University Station, Knoxville, Tn. Phone: (615) 974-5164.

WHAT CAN PSYCHOTHERAPY DO FOR YOU?

When most people have a physical injury, they report to a physician or a hospital as soon as they can. They have no doubt that they should seek care for their injury. However, many people suffer emotional and psychological injuries but do not seek care. Why? Some people may feel that by being treated by a psychotherapist they are labeling themselves as inferior. This could not be further from the truth. Emotional injuries are often more serious, from an overall health standpoint, than physical ones. Many researchers have shown that stress and emotional problems can lower the body's immune response, which makes a person more susceptible to disease. In dentistry, we sometimes see gum disease advance rapidly in a person under extreme stress.

Occasionally, a person will go to a psychotherapist at the request of a friend or a relative. This patient really does not want to go for help and resists the therapy offered. In order to fully benefit from psychotherapy, one must *really want* to be helped. If your friends or relatives suggest psychotherapy to you, decide whether this is something to which you can make a serious commitment. Will you follow instructions? Will you practice? It's up to you.

Psychotherapists can offer many services to help you overcome your fear or phobia. One of the best services they can offer is to really understand your problem from your psychological and emotional perspective. Their insight into psychological processes may enable them to suggest an appropriate method to overcome your fear. They can suggest the appropriate therapy for your individual situation. They can suggest any of the following and can customize that therapy to meet your needs:

- relaxation strategies
- biofeedback training
- hypnosis
- desensitization programs
- group therapy

If you think that you may benefit from the services of a psychologist or a psychiatrist, you owe it to yourself to contact one. Another avenue of help for the dental phobic is the university-based dental fear treatment clinic. This will be discussed in the next chapter.

8

TREATMENT IN A
UNIVERSITY CLINIC

BY TIMOTHY A. SMITH, Ph.D.

This chapter is written by Dr. Timothy Smith, a research psychologist and teacher at the University of Kentucky. Dr. Smith is a professor in the Department of Oral Health Science and also in the Department of Educational and Counseling Psychology. Dr. Smith is a founder of the Dental Fears Treatment Clinic in the College of Dentistry, University of Kentucky, in Lexington. He is the director of a two year research project, "The Formation of an Experimental Treatment Network for Fearful Dental Patients," funded by a national organization, the American Fund for Dental Health. The purpose of this project is to evaluate the dental fear control program (described in Chapter 5).

In the last ten years, several universities and hospitals have begun clinics specializing in the treatment of dental fear. These clincs include those at the universities of Florida (Gainesville), Kentucky (Lexington), and Washington (Seattle), Mount Sinai Hospital in New York City, and Mount Zion Hospital in San Francisco. These clinics are staffed by dentists and psychologists who are trained in how to deal with this difficult problem.

Patients who come to these clinics have often been seen by private-practice dentists who have tried to help them. When these dentists think that special care is needed, they refer them to the fear treatment clinic. Quite often the patients' dental fear is accompanied by other problems, such as fear of going out in public (agoraphobia), allergic reactions to anesthetics, and failure to get numb. The patient may need the services of an anesthesiologist, oral surgeon, or periodontist in addition to the general dentist and psychologist. At a university all of these specialists are available and can coordinate their care.

At the University of Kentucky's Dental Fears Clinic, patients initially encounter a psychologist. They talk about their dental experiences, good and bad, and their emotional reactions to them. They take a battery of tests similar to the ones described in Chapter 5, and in addition complete tests selected to help understand their particular problem.

The first task is to identify the patient's problem and to make a treatment plan for the problem. Often patients are unable to calmly enter a dental clinic and be examined, so the first task is for the psychologist to deal with this anxiety. If the patient does not fear a dental examination, this is usually completed before a treatment plan is developed. In any case, no treatment is attempted unless the patient is comfortable and ready to deal with the stress. Usually the psychologist works with the patient for several appointments before dental treatment (as distinguished from dental examination) is attempted. Patients are taught relaxation methods such as guided imagery and paced breathing and they are instructed to practice them at home with the help of an audiotape. These exercises are then rehearsed in a dental clinic without the presence of a dentist or other personnel. The psychologist guides the patient, who is actually sitting in a dental chair, to imagine the dental appointment taking place. The psychologist then cues the patient to practice the relaxation skills during this simulated dental appointment. An audiotape can be made during this session so that the patient can review it at home and again practice relaxing during a dental appointment.

During the early dental appointments, the psychologist accompanies the patient to help him or her employ the relaxation strategies they have practiced. The psychologist acts as a coach, prompting the patient to use his or her skills when appropriate. The psychologist often monitors vital signs such as pulse, skin temperature, and muscle tension to determine when the patient is getting too tense, so that a rest break can be taken to relax the patient again. The psychologist reminds the dentist of the patient's problems during the appointment so that the dentist can take actions to make the patient comfortable.

Each patient has unique problems which require special care from both the dentist and psychologist. Five cases which have been treated at the University of Kentucky's Dental Fears Clinic illustrate this diversity.

PATIENTS

Stacy was a 36-year-old homemaker and part-time merchandiser with a greeting-card firm. She came to the clinic because of a fear of a reaction to novocaine. Until eight years ago, she had been a regular visitor to the dentist. But after a normal appointment, her face had felt paralyzed and was swollen. Her reaction to what had been a routine injection of novocaine had lasted an hour and was so severe she had to call her husband to drive her home. Since that incident, she had brushed regularly but had not visited the dentist. After a recent visit she had fainted after the injection.

Medically, Stacy had eczema and was allergic to tetracycline. In the past she had been treated for hyperventilation. Drugs scared her; she didn't like being out of control, and she had stopped drinking alcoholic beverages. She considered herself to be a nervous person.

A consultation with a physician showed no medical reasons to withhold regular dental treatment. The psychologist accompanied Stacy to initial appointments, monitoring pulse and skin temperature, which are physiological measures of tension. The psychologist coached Stacy in counting her breaths during the injection in order to distract her and prevent fainting and hyperventilation.

Short, easy dental appointments were scheduled initially. The dentist explained everything, because Stacy feared the unknown and the unexpected. Stacy stayed in the psychologist's office for at least 15 minutes after every dental visit until the anesthetic began to wear off and it was certain no unusual reaction was going to take place.

It was thought that possibly an anesthetic containing epinephrine had caused Stacy's adverse reaction. Epinephrine prolongs the numbing effect of novocaine but may stimulate the person and cause an adverse reaction. Thus an anesthetic (mepivacaine) that did not contain this substance was used in the first three appointments. In the fourth appointment epinephrine was injected and Stacy became very tense, nervous, and her legs shook. This did not occur in following appointments when no epinephrine was injected, and Stacy completed a crown preparation procedure without the psychologist's help. She has now become an enthusiastic recruiter for the clinic.

Arthur was a patient who was massively anxious. The dentist always said it wouldn't hurt, but it did. Even getting his teeth cleaned hurt. About nine years ago Arthur had gum surgery. This procedure was very painful during and after the surgery, and the dentist left town without giving him any postoperative care. It was three months after surgery before his mouth felt normal. Arthur had not been to the dentist since that experience.

Arthur was taught some relaxation techniques to use during the dental appointment. His anticipation tension was high during the examination. He felt great relief when the light was pulled away.

At the next appointment his teeth were cleaned using an ultrasound device and other instruments. The water in his throat made him tense, and he was puckering up and closing his mouth during treatment. Arthur stayed calm from the neck down, but his lips were very tense. More cleaning was done at the following appointment, but Arthur was relaxing more and reported things went better than ever before. Then a filling went even better than past appointments when Arthur had received nitrous oxide. Being told to use his relaxation skills helped get him through the visit. The dentist gave Arthur several injections of anesthetic (injections didn't bother Arthur) so that he was completely numb and felt no pain.

Arthur then was able to complete the next appointment without the assistance of the psychologist. It hadn't been easy, but he had overcome his fear and was able to receive needed dental care.

Claire had seen an article in the newspaper about the University of Kentucky's Dental Fear Clinic. She had trouble getting numb, often needing two injections. She had many fillings done, and even though she was injected, it hurt. She often felt out of control and smothered. She wanted to take care of her teeth but had visions of the dentist yelling at her. Her teeth needed cleaning, and she hadn't chewed on her right side for six months. She said she would rather have a baby than go to the dentist.

Claire rehearsed some relaxation techniques she had learned in a Lamaze childbirth class. At her first appointment she was very tense. It was discovered that she also gagged easily. After the examination, a cleaning was scheduled so that Claire could get accustomed to the dental clinic and to the dentist before something more difficult was scheduled. It also gave Claire a chance to practice her relaxation skills. When a filling was attempted, the dentist explained every step and showed her what was happening in her mouth. This seemed to help a great deal.

Before the next appointment, Claire recounted a dream she had recently had. She was at the dentist's and all the soccer parents had come to watch her. She was tense and required two heavier-than-usual injections. She reported that she felt no pain and had concentrated on breathing and images. She liked the dentist's communicating and explaining things. She said that it was the first dental appointment in which she didn't feel anything or break down.

After her series of appointments was completed, Claire said that it was the first time she had gone to the dentist and not had a painful experience.

Elaine was referred to the clinic by Dr. Kroeger. She had been hospitalized for mental problems in the past and was seeing a hypnotherapist regularly. She was very distrustful of medical and dental personnel and was afraid of panic attacks. She carried a chip-on-the-shoulder attitude. In the past, she had completed extensive dental work but had no memories of going to the dentist. She blocked out memories of medical situations, even having no recollection of her son's being born, including the city where it took place. Twice she had wandered out of dental offices during treatment and gotten lost, once being picked up by the police. She had brought a small clown doll with her to keep her company (Elaine was 39 years old.)

On entering the dental clinic, Elaine acted completely suprised to see dental equipment there, and tried to flee. During the dental examination she appeared extremely frightened, her pupils widely dilated. When an assistant suddenly walked in with a tray of instruments, Elaine tried to jump over the chair and escape. Later she referred to the tray as a display of weapons.

The dentist talked to Elaine in a soft voice, proceeding with the examination very slowly. He told Elaine everything he was going to do so that there would be no surprises. On examination she was diagnosed as having severe gum disease with little hope of saving her teeth.

Because of Elaine's severe phobia and history of mental problems, a decision was made to remove her teeth under general anesthesia. Her complete dentures would be constructed over a period of several weeks. The surgery was successful. Elaine kept her follow-up apointments, even though she lived 100 miles away. The denture was completed and delivered to her over a period of three and a half months. The open, accepting attitude of the staff enabled her to come to the appointments without her doll. She was so pleased with the understanding attitude of the personnel that she made an appointment to see a physician in the same building about another health problem.

Lynn was a medical receptionist who was referred by a local dentists because she reacted to local anesthetics by tachycardia; that is, her heart rate jumped to over 150 beats a minute. She had had rheumatic fever as a child, and any physical effort such as aerobics caused thumping in her chest and dizziness. Her cardiologist, though, reported no special change on recent tests and no evidence of any residual rheumatic fever. Lynn was also being treated by an allergist, who reported multiple allergies to penicillin, sulfa, codeine, and various pain relievers. She reacted to everything but a very weak concentration of local anesthetic.

Lynn reported muscle tension, perspiration, and nausea during dental work. When she was young, she had a severe pain reaction when a dentist struck a nerve during drilling. She waited for that to happen again when the dentist was drilling her teeth.

She needed several fillings, so an appointment was scheduled. All the equipment present in the university clinic to treat medical emergencies was shown to Lynn, and it was emphasized that all personnel had CPR (cardiopulmonary resuscitation) training. One hour before the visit, she took a small dose of a tranquilizer. On being seated in the dental chair, she went through the progressive muscle relaxation exercise for five minutes. A weak concentration of anesthetic was prepared for her. During the injection she counted her breaths to maintain her relaxed state. Immediately after the injection, Lynn became very agitated and her heart rate jumped from 105 to 140. She said it felt like "opening a door" and it took her breath away; she felt like she was smothering. After a three-minute break, she was able to continue with the procedure, though she reported little numbing from the weak anesthetic.

At the next appointment, a more concentrated anesthetic was used, though it was not fully concentrated. Lynn did not react adversely and reported not feeling any pain. The strength of the anesthetic was gradually increased so that Lynn was able to eventually tolerate a full-strength injection, and to skip the tranquilizer before the appointment. She became so comfortable with dental treatment that she sometimes fell asleep during treatment.

LESSONS TO BE LEARNED
FROM THESE PATIENTS

People who are anxious and fearful about dentistry can learn three important lessons from these patients.

First, many people are fearful because of the problems they have with dental anesthetics. Claire never really got numb with a standard dose and so dental treatment always hurt. Some people need more than a normal dose of anesthetic but don't get it or ask for it, and so they have a real reason to be afraid of dentistry.

On the other hand, Stacy and Lynn had severe reactions to anesthetics and so were afraid of going to the dentist for that reason. Allergies are a common condition, and it would be unusual if some people were not allergic to dental substances. These people, too, have a real reason to be nervous about going to the dentist.

Patients should insist that the dentist give them enough anesthetic so that they feel no pain. They also should insist that the dentist use an anesthetic (out of the many available) which will not adversely affect them. A dose of anesthetic costs between 10 and 20 cents; an additional one or two shots will not raise the cost of treatment significantly.

Second, Stacy, Arthur, and Claire illustrate that learning how to use relaxation skills in the dental office takes time. It is relatively easy to relax while sitting at home in an easy chair, but not so easy when someone is drilling on one of your teeth. You can't just do these exercises for the first time in the dental chair and expect them to work. It is necessary to rehearse at home and be willing to endure some problems in early dental visits. While the capsule descriptions of these patients imply that overcoming their dental fear was easy for them, the reverse is true. All these patients are to be commended for their courage, perseverance, and effort.

Third, all of them, especially Lynn and Elaine, show that for some patients a dental fear treatment clinic is the best place for treatment. All benefited from the help of a psychologist in overcoming their fear. Lynn needed the close proximity to complex life support equipment and skilled staff before she could safely try to deal with her allergy problem. Elaine needed a general dentist, psychologist, anesthesiologist, prosthodontist (denture specialist), and oral surgeon to complete her treatment plan. At the university clinic, all these personnel were available so that treatment could be coordinated efficiently. A dental fear treatment clinic can expertly handle patients with complex psychological and dental problems.

9

HOW MEDICATION CAN HELP

Although most patients can tolerate a dental procedure with only the use of a local anesthetic, some patients need stronger medication. An extremely upsetting dental experience may be so deeply ingrained in a patient's memory that he or she feels he cannot get through a procedure without some extra help. I have seen patients who, after initially requesting nitrous oxide, gradually wean themselves off this sedation as their confidence level in themselves and in the dentist increases. In this chapter I will explain some of the options available to patients to provide drug-induced relaxation.

LOCAL ANESTHETICS

Local anesthetics are a class of drugs that normally do not produce relaxation. Instead, they block the pain impulse in a specific area. These are commonly referred to as *novocaine; Novocain*™ is a brand name of a type of a local anesthetic and has not been used in dentistry in many years. Lidocaine and mepivacaine are the two local anesthetics used predominantly in dentistry today. These can provide two to three hours of numbness. Bupivacaine, a long-acting local anesthetic, can provide several hours of numbness and can be used after an extensive procedure to prolong the pain control.

Some fearful patients have concerns about local anesthetics. One concern is tolerance. Some patients claim they have developed a tolerance for local anesthetics, because they always feel pain regardless of the number of injections. Some patients describe this tolerance as an "allergy." What they mean is that they feel their body no longer responds to the drug. While occasionally a patient may have a physical problem (such as dense bone), most of these patients who claim resistance to local anesthetics are extremely fearful and have programmed their minds to interpret any sensation as pain. After catharsis and relaxation training (as in the dental fear control program described in Chapter 5), they usually have no problem in becoming numb. Almost universally, they remark with surprise that they cannot believe the drilling did not hurt.

On the other hand, I have treated a few individuals who did not assume responsibility for their fear, were unwilling to go through the fear control program, and fully expected a lot of pain during treatment. I remember one such individual who, a few years ago, had a toothache. Madge was in severe pain when she came to the office. For the two or three days preceding the appointment, she thought about pain during treatment. She expected the treatment to hurt, she knew it would be terrible, and she was not disappointed. Despite repeated injections, Madge still perceived pain during the drilling. Although Madge represents a very unusual and unique case, she serves as a good example of how important it is for the patient to participate in controlling his or her own fear through relaxation training or other methods.

Other patients report an allergic reaction to novocaine because after the injection, they become short of breath, feel tingling sensations, and feel a rapid and strong heartbeat. Typically, these symptoms in fearful patients are the result of the chemicals produced inside their own bodies by the fear response. If a patient is thoroughly relaxed during the injection, these reactions should be minimized. A true drug-induced allergy to a local anesthetic is extremely rare. This true allergy would involve some or all of the following signs: a rash over the body, itching, swelling, weak pulse, and lowered blood pressure. However, a patient reporting a history of such an episode should be taken seriously and should be tested by a physician who specializes in allergy.

For those patients who feel they have a resistance to local anesthetics and who always feel pain during drilling, I sometimes use a special injection in addition to the normal shot of local anesthetic: the periodontal ligament (PDL) injection. With this injection, the anesthetic solution is deposited near the side of the root of the tooth and, with pressure, is directed to the tip of the root where the nerve enters the tooth. This injection, when combined with the normal injection technique, provides profound numbness, in my experience, about 99 percent of the time. Many dentists I have met also report the same successful results with this dual technique. Sometimes after a PDL injection, you may experience soreness in the gum tissue near the site of the injection. This normally disappears within a few days.

If the PDL technique is used alone, the numbness usually does not spread to the soft tissue (lips, tongue, cheek). This can be advantageous if you have to speak soon after leaving the office. It can also help if you cannot tolerate the idea of numbness (which, to a degree, represents some loss of control). However, the PDL technique by itself is not as predictable in producing profound numbness as the conventional method.

TRANQUILIZERS

One method of providing relaxation is to take a pill before the procedure. These drugs are usually tranquilizers, which produce relaxation in the same center of the brain where the natural relaxation response occurs. You take these pills usually 30 to 60 minutes before the appointment. The major disadvantage of this method is the drowsiness when you leave the office. Someone must accompany you to the office to drive you home. These drugs can linger in the body for up to 48 hours afterward.

However, for some patients, this method may help significantly and may be combined with the use of nitrous oxide sedation for effective relaxation. These medications should be taken only with the dentist's supervision. Certain conditions, such as pregnancy, may rule out this option. Check with your dentist.

NITROUS OXIDE-OXYGEN CONSCIOUS SEDATION

This technique is often referred to as "laughing gas" and may be feared because of that label. Nitrous oxide, if used reasonably, does not make people laugh or embarrass themselves. Although it is a gas, this term may lead people to think of a lethal gas chamber.

Nitrous oxide sedation can provide welcome additional relaxation for those patients who feel they need it. Its major advantage is that the patient leaves the office without drowsiness and can drive home. In today's busy society, that advantage makes this method selected more often than other techniques that cause lingering drowsiness.

One aspect of this method that some fearful patients do not like is that it causes a certain loss of control. A person under this sedation may feel floaty or tingly. This sensation may bother some people. However, most sedation machines can be regulated to decrease the level of sedation to fit the individual's needs.

Nitrous oxide sedation is given simultaneously with oxygen. These two vapors are breathed together through a nasal mask that fits snugly over the nose. If the amount of nitrous oxide is increased, you will feel more deeply relaxed. You can always signal to the dentist if you feel too deeply

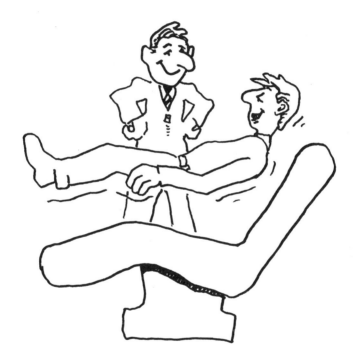

"Dr. Jones, I think I've had enough nitrous oxide, now."

relaxed. The safety record for nitrous oxide use in dental offices is extremely good. Many patients remark that it helps them tremendously in the initial stages of their dental treatment. Fearful patients sometimes use nitrous oxide along with headphones playing the relaxation tapes during their first few appointments. As their trust level increases and as their skills in natural relaxation exercises develop, these patients often tell me they no longer need nitrous oxide.

Some patients with severe, uncontrolled fear will not benefit from nitrous oxide because their internal stress response overrides its relaxation effect. Patients who are dependent on drugs (such as alcoholics) will typically not benefit from this method. Patients who are pregnant or who have certain other medical conditions should not use nitrous oxide. However, since it is extremely safe, nitrous oxide sedation can be used for most patients. Consult with your dentist regarding any medical condition you have before beginning treatment.

In general, nitrous oxide provides a wonderful feeling of well-being. Patients are aware of what is going on around them but they are far less concerned about it. By breathing the pleasant aroma through the nosepiece, patients are able to have their dental treatment accomplished with safety and in comfort and relaxation. The following are the major effects felt by patients under nitrous oxide:

- tingling sensation in the fingers, legs, toes, and lips
- sensation of warmth
- dizzy feeling
- possible sweating
- a feeling of happiness (euphoria)

In some deeper stages of nitrous oxide administration, the patient may dream, become sleepy, or feel nauseated. These conditions may be reversed by decreasing the concentration of nitrous oxide.

Although natural relaxation methods and nitrous oxide will help most patients, a few may need deeper relaxation provided by intravenous sedation.

INTRAVENOUS SEDATION

Intravenous sedation provides rapid, deep relaxation by drugs injected directly into the bloodstream. Two main types are available: conscious and unconscious. In both techniques, the drug is usually injected into a vein in the arm with an intravenous saline drip being attached. In the conscious technique, the patient is groggy and is usually more deeply sedated than with nitrous oxide. In the unconscious technique, the patient is completely asleep, although there are various levels of sedation even at this stage.

Obviously, the major disadvantage is recovery time. You may need anywhere from 30 minutes to a few hours to regain enough composure to leave the office. Someone will have to drive you home. Risk factors are also a consideration whenever intravenous sedation is used. Although very rare, deaths have been reported when a patient was rendered unconscious under intravenous sedation in the dental office. The safety record of oral surgeons using outpatient intravenous sedation has been remarkably excellent, far surpassing that of hospitals in this regard.

The major advantage, especially with the unconscious method, is that you can have an extensive procedure performed with absolutely no pain. If this technique is used, someone must monitor the patient's vital signs. Because the overhead expense of this sedation can be considerable, a separate fee is usually required for this service.

Some patients want to have all their dental work done while under unconscious sedation. But it is very difficult to achieve excellence in some areas of dentistry in this fashion. Also, the patients' fear is not overcome. Their fear or phobia may still be powerful enough to cause them to continue to avoid the dentist, with the end result being a deteriorated mouth several years hence.

These medications are described to give you some idea of what options you have. Ideally, most patients can provide their own relaxation naturally, which affords them a sense of self-control and a sense of self-confidence. It also increases the chances of fearful patients overcoming their fear and of returning to the office for periodic examination and cleaning.

10

COPING WITH SPECIFIC PROCEDURES AND FEARS

Many patients have a generalized (and often justified) fear of the unknown in the dentist's office. This fear can be intensified in patients with active imaginations. Not knowing what a specific procedure involves can lead some fearful patients to imagine the worst. In this chapter, I will explain some of the basics in most dental procedures which will help you understand why certain things are done. This knowledge should help you feel more comfortable in the dental chair and should help to reduce your fear or phobia.

A form presented in Chapter 5 listed about 30 different dental fears. You may have already reviewed this form. If not, please do, circling any fears you may have and writing down any bad experiences surrounding these fears. In this chapter, these fears will be described in depth and some will be illustrated with case studies. I will explain some coping methods for these fears. You may be creative and formulate some coping strategies yourself. Your own ideas may work well. At the end of the chapter, a self-assessment section is available for your use.

In general, the dental fear control program (Chapter 5) will help a patient cope with each of these fears. Learning progressive muscle relaxation and guided imagery is a prerequisite in dealing with any of these fears or phobias. Desensitization is also useful.

PATIENT ASSERTIVENESS

To many patients, the dentist is like a deity placed high on a pedestal. Thus the patient can feel intimidated. Fearful patients, especially, may not want to tell the dentist that they are in pain or need a break. This lack of assertiveness may result in pain or some other bad experience. *It is your responsibility* to tell the dentist if something hurts or if you want to take a break (to rinse, to breathe, to go to the bathroom). Most dentists truly care about their patients' comfort and are willing to pause during treatment. *It is up to you* to inform the dentist that you want him or her to stop.

But if you need frequent breaks during treatment, you should realize that the fee for treatment may be increased because the procedure will require more of the dentist's time and more overhead (staff salaries, electricity, materials, and so on). You can reduce your dental bills by going through the dental fear control program (Chapter 5) or through a similar program and by following the tips in this chapter. Lower bills represent less time for you in the dental chair — a welcome thought for many fearful patients.

GENERAL TREATMENT RULES

1. Ask for a brief description of what the dentist plans to do. If you know something in the procedure might bother you, explain your concerns. Can this particular aspect of treatment be avoided or altered for you? (Please remember, in order to accomplish excellent technical

dentistry, some procedures cannot be altered.)
2. If you intensely fear a certain procedure, see whether the dentist can introduce it to you slowly and gently, perhaps spreading treatment over several visits.
3. If you begin to feel uncomfortable (for whatever reason), let the dentist and staff know about it at once. Don't wait until you feel overwhelmed. This may cause you not to return for further treatment.
4. Prearrange with the dentist for a signal (such as raising your hand) to indicate you want him to stop or that you are in pain. If you are in pain, *immediately* use this signal to let the dentist know. If the dentist does not stop, be assertive and stop the procedure yourself. Please remember two things here: (1) If you are extremely fearful or phobic and have done nothing to reduce your fear (fear control program, relaxation exercises, psychotherapy), the dentist may have a very difficult time treating you painlessly. (2) Most procedures can be ended by using some type of temporary measure so that the treatment can be performed at a future date. If the dentist is causing pain and says that he has done all he can to prevent it, you can either have the procedure completed or request temporary measures so that you can have the treatment continued at a future appointment. But, in the meantime, if you have not taken any responsibility to reduce your fear level, your emotional state may still be predisposed to feeling pain. You may ask your dentist, at this stage, whether he thinks that nitrous oxide or tranquilizers would help you to further relax.

My staff and I have success in treating fearful and phobic patients without pain 99 percent of the time. Sometimes they feel pressure, a slight sensation, or some discomfort. But I always tell each patient to report any sharp pain immediately and I then stop the procedure. Often, dentists can use a supplementary injection method to provide for profound numbness.

A TYPICAL TREATMENT PROCEDURE

Here's what you can expect during a typical treatment procedure and also what you can do to make it as comfortable as possible for yourself.

Before The Appointment

Don't drink anything with caffeine (coffee, tea, most soft drinks) before your dental visit. Caffeine is a stimulant and it may make you feel nervous, hindering relaxation. Unless you are having a general anesthetic (being put to sleep), eat something before your visit, such as protein or carbohydrate. An empty stomach during your treatment may cause you to feel faint.

About one hour before your visit, practice a relaxation exercise, such as progressive muscle relaxation or guided imagery. Think positive thoughts and become deeply relaxed. Then, allowing yourself plenty of time, drive *slowly* to the dental office. Don't try to arrive on the exact minute of your appointment. If you encounter a traffic delay, you will have to rush and you may be late for your appointment. You will then feel upset when you arrive, which will add to your fear level.

Try to arrive at least 15 minutes early so that you can listen to a relaxation tape before going to the treatment room. If the dental office has a "quiet room" (no dental equipment), that is the ideal place for you to wait and practice the relaxation exercise. Again, think positive thoughts during this time, driving any negative thoughts out of your mind. Expect the best.

As you're escorted to the treatment room, you may notice your body beginning to show signs of the stress response: sweaty palms, rapid heartbeat, and stomach butterflies. Now, you must practice a relaxation exercise to cancel out these fear symptoms. Again, think positive thoughts at this time. Discuss with the dental assistant what procedure(s) will be done and ask whether you can use stereo headphones to listen to your relaxation tape. This will also block out the noise of the drilling. If the dental office does not have headphones, bring your own set.

When the dentist enters the treatment room, he or she may discuss with you some particulars about today's treatment. Now you can mention any fears or concerns you may have. Also decide on what signal you can give to ask the dentist to stop. If the dentist has nitrous oxide available, and you think you'll need it for the injection or for the procedure, ask about it.

The Injection Begins

For many patients, the injection of novocaine is the most feared aspect of the entire procedure, even with today's tiny needles and gentle techniques. Before the dentist begins the injection, place your hands together over the middle of your stomach area. This will help you feel more protected. Also begin to practice guided imagery, moving your mind to a distant beach and concentrating on the waves rolling in and the crystal clear water, instead of the injection. If this is difficult, concentrate on breathing slowly and deeply. This will also help you relax and will make it easier for the dentist to give a gentle injection.

Typically, the first thing the dentist does is to place a swab with an anesthetic cream on the gum at the site of the injection. This cream has a numbing effect on the gum. After 20 to 30 seconds (with the cream), the dentist inserts the needle. The dentist then injects slowly, which allows the novocaine to penetrate gently into the tissues. Although this may seem like it's taking forever, this slow technique results in a gentle injection. During or after the injection, you may notice your heart beating rapidly or a tingly sensation coming over your body. This could be the result of the natural release of adrenaline that accompanies the fear (stress)

response. These sensations may also be caused by the novocaine. If you have these sensations, you should discuss them
with the dentist and you should be monitored until they
disappear, which usually happens in a few minutes. Relaxation exercises will also help you here.

Sometimes you may feel an electric shock during an
injection. This is caused by the needle touching a structure
(usually a nerve). Normally, this does not happen. If it does,
it is no reflection on the technique of the dentist but rather
on the anatomical position of the structures in your mouth.
If the shock should happen on your lower lip, that means
that the nerves of the teeth should be numbed profoundly.

Patients have needle phobia, often fainting at the sight of
any needle. I once treated a highly educated woman (Ph.D.
in science) who had such a phobia. Outwardly appearing
calm and collected, she matter-of-factly told me that she
would pass out at the sight or the thought of a needle. She
told me that it happened frequently. The purpose of her
visit was a routine dental filling. During the visit, I described
my gentle injection technique including use of a topical
cream to numb the surface of the gum prior to injecting.
However, before I was able to perform the injection, she
fainted as she had predicted. She neither saw the needle nor
received the injection before she fainted. Her memory bank
of bad experiences had programmed her behavior and
caused her to faint.

Another needle phobic was a young man who told me
that he routinely fainted at the sight of a needle. I again
reassured him and used a gentle injection technique. He
closed his eyes during the injection and did not faint,
although he did show profuse sweating and rapid
breathing. On his next visit, he was still very fearful. This
time during the injection, I told him that the needle was in
his mouth and he had no pain. I then said that if he had no
pain during this injection, needles couldn't be all so bad,
after all. I wanted him to see the needle in his mouth. After
he agreed to watch, I gave him a mirror and he was sur-

prised to see there was no pain associated with the sight of the needle. After that experience, he no longer had a great fear of needles.

Nitrous oxide sedation is useful in relaxing a needle phobic before an injection. Many phobics report that this helps initially, and, after learning self-relaxation, they no longer need the nitrous oxide for the injection.

Another method is systematic desensitization, both in imagination and in real life. You imagine receiving an injection and then perform a relaxation exercise. After practicing this technique, you gradually do not feel fearful when *imagining* the injection. Then, you can look at an actual syringe, feel it, and examine it. When you feel comfortable with this, you may allow the dentist to place the syringe (with the protective cap covering the needle) in your mouth. In this manner, you are gradually exposed to the feared needle until this fear disappears or is lessened.

Machines providing electrical anesthesia (without needles) are now available but are not totally predictable. With further research, this method may become an excellent anesthetic technique for the needle phobic. Unfortunately, much of the publicity for this method emphasizes the total elimination of the needle in dental practice. This is erroneous. The technique, transcutaneous electrical nerve stimulation (abbreviated t.e.n.s.), offers several advantages: a needleless application, no lingering numbness, and no possiblity of nerve shocks. The patient controls the amount of stimulation by regulating the machine via a handset control. However, this method also has some disadvantages: lack of predictability in producing effective anesthesia (60 percent vs 99 percent with novocaine), a significant waiting time before numbness develops, a possibility of flashing lights in the patient's vision, a learning period for patient and dentist, and mild electrical shocks. The major disadvantage is the time required to wait for the onset of numbness. If nothing happens, the dentist must then give an injection of novocaine and again wait for that to take effect.

The increased time spent in the dental chair may be reflected in the fee.

The Drilling Begins

Most dental procedures involve the drill. Fear of pain during drilling is probably the most common fear. Vivid memories of bad experiences increase the perception of pain, as the gate control theory explains (Chapter 3). You can apply information in Chapter 3 about how you can raise your pain perception threshold here. Your relaxed mental state will definitely help you tolerate the drilling better than if all your bad dental experiences are being replayed in your memory. Remember the examples of Mary and Harriet from Chapter 3? Mary, the fearful patient, had programmed her brain to expect pain and she was not disappointed. Harriet, the relaxed patient, tolerated her procedures well, without any novocaine.

The major method for overcoming this fear is to develop a strong bond of trust with your dentist. You must truly believe that the dentist or staff person will not hurt you intentionally. Accidental pain is always possible, but you must remember that you can stop the procedure by raising your hand or by some other signal.

Obviously, the dentist and staff must be gentle, caring, and respond to your signal to stop. If I encounter a patient who is very concerned about being hurt during drilling, I try to erase this fear as quickly as possible. I make three statements to the patient: (1) If you want a break during the drilling, please raise your hand to stop the procedure — this gives you control over the situation. (2) I can produce a profound numbness in your tooth that will be effective. (3) If the drilling produces any pain, I will stop and use an additional technique that will numb your tooth completely. My confidence in these statements helps reassure the patient.

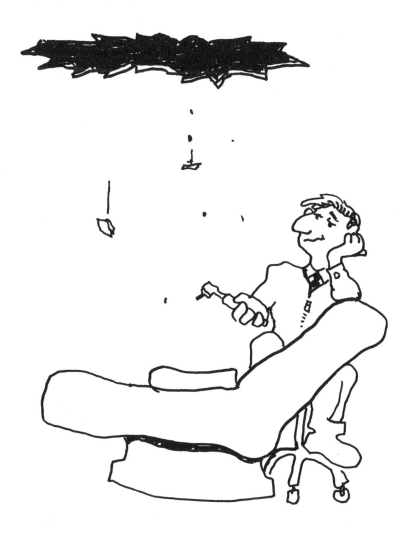

"Now, that didn't hurt very much, did it?"

In preparing for the drilling, again place your hands over your stomach. Review with the dentist your signal to stop drilling. Plan to use your headphones, since blocking out the sound of the drill helps significantly. Try your best to hold very still during the drilling; if you make a quick movement, such as jerking your head, the high-speed drill may do something undesirable. Dentistry is a precise science. The dentist needs all the help you can give in order to provide you with excellent results. If you find you simply cannot sit still for the procedure, the dentist may elect to place a temporary filling and postpone the treatment. However, the fee for the appointment may reflect the total time of service given to you and not simply the temporary restoration.

If you feel you need to rinse or take a break, ask the dentist whether this is possible. This may help you get through the procedure, especially if it is lengthy.

Use your headphones, your mental relaxation exercises, and, if necessary, nitrous oxide. If you have trouble using imagery or progressive relaxation, try distracting yourself. Look at a ceiling tile. (Some dental offices have pictures on the ceiling.) Count from 100 back to zero. Above all, think positive thoughts and drive any negative thoughts out of your mind.

At the completion of the drilling, take a moment or two to sit in the chair (in the upright position) to regain your composure and equilibrium. At this time you can thank the dentist and assistant for being gentle and for taking the time and effort to be caring enough to make the procedure comfortable for you. Dentists and staff members appreciate hearing a thank you, and it reinforces their positive feelings toward you. It also motivates them to be gentle with you the next time. The dentist also appreciates your referrals of your friends and relatives.

As you get out of the dental chair, take a few steps to see how you feel. If you feel weak or faint, tell the dental assistant and sit back in the chair. Don't try to wish away these feelings. You may need to breathe oxygen for a few minutes.

As you leave the office, you should feel proud of yourself for having had the courage to tolerate the procedure. You should remember all the positive aspects of your dental visit and concentrate on these. If something didn't go as well as you would have liked, don't worry about it. You'll do better next time. Concentrate on your successes.

OTHER TREATMENT PROCEDURES

Impressions

Impressions are made when crowns, fixed bridges, dentures, and other appliances are to be constructed. Many people worry about gagging during an impression. Gagging usually occurs because they fear the soft impression material will run down their throat and cause them to choke. Sometimes, if the material is runny, this may be a valid concern. Most of the time, however, the impression material will not run down the throat.

What can you do to minimize gagging? Because gagging is essentially a contraction of muscles, any effort on your part to relax your muscles will reduce the chance of gagging. Use progressive muscle relaxation for 10 to 15 minutes before this session, concentrating on the muscles of the head and neck region. During the impression, raise your leg off the chair and suspend it in air. It's hard to tense two different muscles in the body at the same time. Also, concentrate on blowing air through your nose during the impression. Using guided imagery will help distract you. Nitrous oxide sedation also helps to reduce the gag reflex. A recent study indicated that eating some salt immediately before the impression was helpful in reducing gagging.

X Rays

For some people, X rays can also cause gagging. Use the same steps outlined above. Sometimes the edges of the X-ray film can seem rough. If the film is bent slightly to conform better to the shape of your mouth, this may be more comfortable for you. Some patients also have a fear of radiation exposure during X rays. While there is some radiation exposure, the use of modern equipment (such as high-speed X-ray film, X-ray machines with shorter exposure times, and protective lead shields that the patient wears) helps minimize this radiation.

Crown Preparation

When a tooth is prepared for a crown (cap), the dentist must take time to produce the desired result. This may mean a visit of over one hour for a single tooth. If you have trouble opening your mouth for a long period of time, you might request the dentist to give you a rubber bite block that will prop open your mouth and may make this part easier for you. Impressions are usually made at this appointment. It is very important for you to remain still during these impressions, since they must be absolutely precise in order to make an excellent crown.

When the crown is cemented, if the tooth is particularly sensitive, you may request a local anesthetic. However, this may make it difficult for the dentist to be sure that the crown is in harmony with the rest of your bite. Usually no anesthetic is required during the fitting. However, the tooth must be dried prior to cementation, which may cause sensitivity. Here you may want to request numbness.

Endodontics (Root Canal Therapy)

This is a treatment feared by many people. It is frequently the butt of jokes in the media which intensifies the negative image of root canals. Normally, a tooth is very sick when a root canal procedure has to be performed. The more abscessed the tooth is, the more difficult the procedure. Regular checkups can help the dentist to detect and treat small cavities before they grow larger and require root canal therapy.

In root canal treatment, a rubber protective mask, called a rubber dam, is used for several reasons. Because it encloses the mouth, it can be feared by some patients who have claustrophobia, an abnormal fear of being closed in. Reassurance by the dentist and staff helps in this situation.

At times during a root canal session, you may experience pain. If this happens, you should signal to the dentist and the dentist should stop to inject more anesthetic. Techniques are available today to produce profound numbness so that procedures like root canals can be performed without pain.

If a root canal is being performed on a tooth that has a dead nerve, you may not need an anesthetic because you may not have any pain.

Occasionally you may have pain. The dentist, anticipating this, may ask you if you would like additional novocaine to last for some time after you leave the office. Available today are long-acting local anesthetics to provide excellent postoperative pain control.

Periodontics (Scalings and Gum Surgery)

These procedures are also feared by many people. However, like root canal therapy, they save teeth. And having natural teeth is much better than wearing dentures.

Deep scaling procedures are designed to remove hard deposits of tartar from the roots of teeth. Since the roots are covered with only a thin protective layer, they may pick up sensations more readily than the enamel that coats the exposed part of the tooth. For this reason, you may prefer to be numb for this procedure. Also, the better you floss and brush your gums, the tougher they will become and thus be less sensitive during these procedures.

Gum surgery can be an elaborate procedure for several reasons. Again, concentrate on the benefits of saving your teeth: chewing, smiling, laughing, speaking, and esthetics. Sometimes after treatment, the roots of the teeth will be exposed, causing sensitivity. Various methods can be used (such as desensitizing medications and bonding) to minimize this.

Oral Surgery Procedures

Any surgical procedure in the mouth may result in postoperative pain. Pain medications and long-acting numbing methods can provide effective relief.

Extensive oral surgical procedures may require a general anesthetic. This means being put to sleep during the procedure. However, some fearful patients want a general anesthetic for a minor oral surgical procedure that could be performed with novocaine alone. You should realize that when you have a general anesthetic, you assume a risk while you are unconscious.

If you have prolonged pain after a surgical procedure, you should contact your dentist, since this could indicate an infection or some other problem. Most dentists are more than willing to provide follow-up care for any difficulties you might have.

Fillings

Fear of the injection and fear of pain during the drilling are the two most common concerns when fillings are done. Some recent advances in filling technology have reduced the need for injections and drilling.

One such development is called bonding which involves making the front teeth whiter and more esthetic. In this

technique, a porcelain-like material is adapted to the surface of the tooth to produce a desired shape and color. This
material is attached to the tooth by an extremely durable
adhesive process. Bonding often requires minimal drilling,
which means that the injection is not needed. At times,
however, the edge of the fillings must be polished near the
root surface. This can produce pain. In this instance, a local
anesthetic may be necessary.

Another development is a liquid form of decay removal.
In this method, a chemical solution is sprayed into the
decayed area of a tooth. After several minutes, the decay is
easily removed with the spray. Unfortunately, much of the
publicity surrounding this technique leads one to believe
that no drilling and no injections are necessary. To the
contrary, an injection and drilling are required for most
quality restorations. To provide a quality restoration, the
dentist must shape the tooth in a precise manner. This
drilling and shaping will usually produce pain, especially in
fearful patients, if no local anesthetic is used. However, this
liquid does remove decay, even though the time required is
much longer than if done with a drill. The time and
expense of the system are usually reflected in the fee for the
procedure.

OTHER FEARS

Fear of Being Criticized

Many dental phobics regard this fear as a major factor in
avoiding the dentist. As they continue to avoid seeing the
dentist and as their mouths deteriorate, they worry that they
will be scolded by the dentist or staff for their neglect.

Dentists must realize that for a dental phobic, his or her
phobia is as crippling as two broken legs in keeping him
away from a dental office. If the dentist and staff are critical

of the dental phobic, he has the option of selecting a new dentist. When calling for the intial appointment, however, the patient should explain his fear of being criticized so that the dentist and staff understand this fear ahead of time.

In our office, my staff and I try to emphasize the positive aspects of the dental phobic's mouth. We try to congratulate the patient on having made the courageous decision to visit the dentist. The patient knows his mouth is in terrible shape and he may not want to hear that at the first appointment. Many times a patient has remarked to me that this was the first time anybody had anything good to say about his mouth.

Fear of Embarrassing the Dentist and Staff

Closely associated with the preceding fear is the fear of embarrassing the dentist and staff. The patient often thinks that his mouth is probably the worst mouth in the world. He or she imagines that the dentist has never seen such a mouth and will be shocked. Again, the patient fears being embarrassed and possibly being criticized.

The dentist and staff have typically seen many patients with deteriorated mouths. You are not the first and probably not the worst. One of the most interesting observations I have made in my dental practice is that almost every highly fearful or phobic patient is extremely relieved to hear that his or her mouth is not one of the worst that I have seen. If the dentist and staff are truly caring and have empathy with you, they will not be embarrassed and they will not criticize you.

Fear of Being Ignored

Sometimes, the dentist and assistant will carry on a conversation, unintentionally excluding you. If the you are particularly sensitive to this (many people under extreme stress become hypersensitive), you may feel offended. With fingers and instruments inside your mouth, it is difficult for you to respond in this situation. At times, the dentist and staff need to communicate in technical terms. They are doing this to maximize efficiency and to complete the procedure — not to exclude you.

As with any other fear, you must inform the dentist and staff about this fear before treatment begins.

Fear of Extraction of a Tooth

Many patients fear the extraction of a tooth. For men, this can subconsciously symbolize the partial loss of virility. This subconscious fear can make a person refuse an extraction when the tooth cannot be saved. Many fearful patients who have avoided the dentist for a long time think their teeth have deteriorated so badly they will require extraction. Fearing the consequences of extractions, they continue to avoid dental care. I frequently see a grateful smile of relief when I tell a patient his or her teeth can be restored and saved. Patients may also fear extractions because extractions may symbolize the aging process and a worsened physical appearance.

Many teeth today can be saved. However, some must be extracted. With the development of dental implants, patients may have options other than a full denture when they lose all their teeth.

Some patients fear pain during an extraction. Normally, it is fairly easy to deaden the tooth for an extraction. Often only pressure only is felt during an extraction. However, depending on the pain threshold and pain perception, this pressure sensation may be interpreted as painful. Some wisdom teeth and other situations do not lend themselves to a simple extraction routine and may require a surgical approach. In some cases, a general anesthetic may be indicated.

Fear of the Fee

Some patients, even wealthy ones, will be afraid of this. In past instances, they may have thought they were "overcharged," not understanding why they were charged for a certain procedure. They may not have learned the relationship between excellence and cost of services. Excellence costs money. Patients may not understand quality of dentistry from a technical aspect (such as the dentist taking continuing education courses, making meticulous impressions, developing a harmonious fit of the teeth, and monitoring for gum disease). Once patients understand the value of a healthy mouth, they may appreciate the value of high-quality dentistry. Naturally, the fearful patient who has a mouthful of decayed teeth may think it will cost many dollars to restore his or her mouth. And he may be correct, especially if he wants a good job. In most cases, when the fearful patient realizes how caring and gentle the dentist and staff are and how much time they spend trying to make him comfortable, the value of excellent dentistry may be apparent and the fee may seem well worth every dollar.

Because many fearful patients have not visited a dentist in 5-10 years or longer, they may have memories of dental fees from their last dental visit many years ago. When they are informed about the current fees for treatment, they experience "sticker shock." This is equivalent to several years ago when car prices seemed to skyrocket rather rapidly. The dental phobic may need some time to accept the reality that his or her mouth deserves the best dentistry and that it may cost a substantial amount. It may also take some time to be comfortable with the dentist and staff in order to develop enough trust to allow them to restore his mouth. For some people, this time period may be only a few weeks; for others it may be years.

Fear of the Results of the Examination

For fearful and phobic patients who have avoided the dentist for years, fear of frequent trips to the dental office is a realistic concern.

Dentistry today, however, is sophisticated compared to 20 or even 10 years ago. Many procedures can be streamlined for patient comfort. Multiple treatments can be done in one session. Discuss this fear with your dentist to learn how your treatment can be accomplished with minimal distress for you.

Fear of the Dentist Slipping

This fear can be magnified by an active imagination. If you had a past bad experience where the dentist did make a mistake, you may be justified in being concerned that a mistake may happen again. However, many people who have this fear have acquired it from hearsay. Most dentists are highly skilled professionals who dedicate themselves to caring for patients. You should understand that a slip happens very rarely and that you can help prevent it by raising your hand if discomfort occurs rather than sudenly jerking your head.

Fear of Gagging

Since the gag reflex is essentially a protective mechanism, this can be considered a reasonable concern. However, this response can vary in intensity from a mild gag reflex to an overpowering rejection of anything approaching the mouth. Most of the time, gagging is caused by fear of choking on or of swallowing a foreign object.

Years ago, a patient new to my practice said she had a strong gag reflex and had been critized by her former

dentist. After she became my patient, she gradually over-
came this fear. Once she discovered that dentistry could be
performed gently, she "forgot" about her psychologically
related gag reflex. She had many crowns and fixed bridges
successfully completed and was very surprised that she
never gagged.

Suggestions for coping with this fear have been discussed
earlier in this chapter in the section on impressions.

Fear of the Sound of Drilling

The sound of the drill may revive memories of painful
experiences. These memories may contribute to an
increased awareness of pain. Headphones with music help
to block out the noise. You may find a hand control useful to
regulate the volume, increasing it as the sound of the drilling increases. Some patients prefer to listen to the relaxation
audiotapes while other prefer their own musical tapes or the
radio.

Fear of a Sharp Instrument Being Stuck Inside a Sensitive Part of the Tooth

This may seem to be a minor concern. However, some
patients feel very strongly about this aspect of an examination. Some patients will vividly describe how their former
dentist would stick "that little pick" into their tooth so far
that it would cause considerable pain. A dentist can use this
instrument, called an explorer, gently and carefully so that
you will not experience pain. Tell your dentist about this
fear so he will be careful during your exam.

Fear of Being Confined in a Small Space

Claustrophobia is not a common fear in dental patients. It
may indicate an additional psychological problem that may

need treatment by a psychotherapist. Some normal-sized treatment rooms can seem tiny to this type of patient. Again, express this fear to your dentist. You may need to take a break once in a while to leave the room. Distraction through guided imagery will also help.

Fear of Bleeding

This fear may be justified; extensive bleeding is a serious matter. But this fear may become blown out of proportion and grow into a phobia. Some patients fear bleeding after an extraction or after gum surgery. If you have no history of bleeding or clotting problems, you should understand that excessive bleeding in the mouth is rare. If you do have a bleeding problem, however, appropriate precautions should be taken by the dentist.

Fear of Numbness

Many people dislike the lingering feeling of numbness when the appointment is finished. On the other hand, many fearful patients are reassured by the numb feeling in that they will not experience pain during drilling. Other patients have a phobia about losing control over themselves which they associate with the numb feeling. This may indicate additional psychological problems.

One patient was referred to our office by a psychologist who discovered the patient had dental phobia. She also had a severe phobia about losing control through the numb feeling. She did not want nitrous oxide or intravenous sedation. I used the PDL technique (described in Chapter 9) that did not produce any numbness of the lips or tongue. She tolerated this well enough to have her mouth restored.

Fear of Extreme Pain After The Numbness Has Worn Off

A person with this fear usually has had prior bad experiences. The dentist can use a special long-acting local anesthetic to provide hours of pain relief in this situation. Ask your dentist to give you such an anesthetic (the generic name is bupivacaine). Other oral pain medications can be prescribed.

Fear of Swelling

The dentist has certain medications available to decrease postoperative swelling. An ice bag applied to the area of surgery will also help reduce swelling. Apply the ice as directed by your dentist.

Fear of Invasion (Violation of Self)

A study has shown that most people feel their "self" is located in the head area. It is normal to protect the face and head from sudden danger. However, an extreme fear of invasion into the mouth may indicate an underlying psychological problem. Patients with this problem may be difficult to treat, misinterpret the dentist's actions, and feel abused. These patients may need the help of a psychotherapist.

Fear of Dentistry in General

Distress and fear can cloud the memory. Some people may not be able to remember any specific instance when they were hurt, but may have vague memories of pain. Combined with hearsay and media influence, this may give them an uneasy feeling about dentistry in general. A trusting relationship with the dentist and staff will help eliminate this fear. Try to remember what caused your fear. If you can identify your fear, chances are good that your dentist can help you.

One further note: Don't be surprised if you see your dentist and dental assistant wearing gloves and masks during treatment. This may seem somewhat scary to you at first. Understand that it is an excellent method for controlling the spread of disease. These preventive measures are for the protection of you, the patient, as well as for the dentist and staff. This means that you will not receive any germs from any prior patients and that your germs will not be transferred to anyone else. Everyone has germs in the mouth. You should feel more secure, knowing that your dental office tries to be as sterile as possible.

If you have a fear of any other dental procedure, tell your dentist or assistant about this fear. He or she can then explain to you his methods and can reassure you about your fear. This information should provide you with knowledge that will enable you to become more confident in your dental visits. Sometimes, patients need extra help involving systematic desensitization. This is the topic of the next chapter.

SELF-ASSESSMENT

1. What are my greatest fears?

   * _____
   * _____
   * _____
   * _____

2. Have I told my dentist and his or her staff about these fears?
3. Have I learned the relaxation exercises of guided imagery and progressive muscle relaxation?

4. Have I tried systematic desensitization?
5. Outline for my own personal strategy to overcome my fears:

- _____

- _____

- _____

- _____

- _____

11

PRACTICING DESENSITIZATION

In 1958 Dr. Joseph Wolpe described a technique he found to be effective in treating people with phobias. This technique, called systematic desensitization, has been used extensively by psychologists and psychiatrists for the past 30 years with tremendous success in helping phobic individuals. This technique was described as part of the dental fear control program in Chapter 5. In this chapter, we will take a more detailed look at this excellent method. Systematic desensitization is a means of reducing a person's fear by gradually exposing the person to the feared object or situation. Some effective remedies for common dental fears will be presented. You will also be shown how to structure an individualized method to counteract your specific fear(s).

In systematic desensitization, the object is to train the mind to substitute relaxation for anxiety in response to the feared situation. The secret behind this method is learning to produce deep relaxation (through any of the relaxation exercises described in Chapters 4 and 6) and having a strong desire to succeed in overcoming fear. By training your "automatic" nervous system to produce deep relaxation, *at your command,* you can reprogram your mind and eliminate your fears.

If you are highly motivated, you may accomplish great results with the exercises in this chapter. However, you may also benefit significantly from the help of a support person or a behavioral specialist such as a psychologist or a psychiatrist. The value of psychotherapy has been described in Chapter 7. A support person may also be a great boost for your determination. Knowing that someone is behind you, encouraging your efforts, is motivating.

Look at John's fear of dogs, as an example. At first, John learns to deeply relax. Then he imagines the sight and sound of a dog in various scenes, while relaxing at each scene. After becoming confident in these imaginary exercises, John is brought into a room where a live dog is positioned about 50 feet away from him. He immediately relaxes himself deeply. Slowly, he is moved closer to the dog, a few feet at a time, relaxing after each step. This may be repeated, over a period of time ranging from a few days to weeks or longer, until John can actually pet the dog without fear.

PRINCIPLES OF DESENSITIZATION

- The key idea is prolonged exposure to the feared object or activity.
- Repeat this exposure daily, weekly, and monthly until the fear or anxiety diminishes.
- Ingrain the confidence of success into your memory.
- Don't push yourself too rapidly — move at your own pace. Your support person or therapist should also respect your pace.
- Periodically rate your progress, noting gradual improvement.
- Never prevent yourself from leaving the feared situation if you become extremely anxious. This may cause a panic

attack, an extreme physical response including pounding heart, rapid breathing, and a sense of impending doom.

Important: If you have any heart problems, high blood pressure, or a medical condition requiring medication, you should consult with your physician before attempting to become deeply aroused by any feared situation.

Let's consider another example of a phobia that is almost universally shared: the fear of public speaking. Jane was promoted to a position that required her to occasionally give a presentation in front of an audience of her peers. In the past, she had become extremely fearful in this situation to the point where she felt her heart beating so rapidly that she felt it pounding through her blouse. Her mouth became dry and she had much difficulty in speaking.

In her therapy, Jane first learned progressive muscle relaxation. After weeks of practicing, she eventually became skilled in this method. She then learned as many useful speaking techniques as she could and practiced them. Finally, she practiced imagining herself being introduced and successfully giving a speech. She fashioned a fear ladder beginning with the least offensive scene and concluding

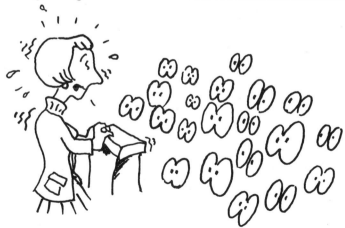

Fear Of Public Speaking

with the scene she feared the most (staring out into the large audience). She practiced imagining the scenes over and over again, following each with deep relaxation.

She then practiced giving speeches to her support person and then to a small group of friends. *Gradually,* she built up enough confidence to give a presentation to a large group. After *repeated exposure* to the public speaking situation, Jane's phobia lessened to the point where it no longer had a paralyzing grip on her.

And so can you have similiar success with your fears or phobias about dentistry. By following these same principles, you can overcome your problems the way countless other people overcome their phobias on a daily basis.

What follows are examples of dental fear desensitization exercises. If your fear is one of the following, you may use it or adapt it to your situation. If you have a dental fear not included here, you can create your own desensitization approach or work with your therapist who will help you.

NEEDLE PHOBIA DESENSITIZATION

This is a major fear in dentistry. Figure 12 illustrates two syringes with dental needles. Look at these during your exercise.

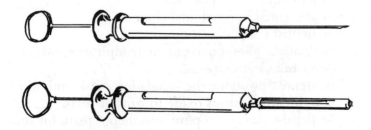

Dental Needles

Fig. 12

Exercise No. 1. Visualize each of the following scenes. Then practice either progressive muscle relaxation or guided imagery until you can visualize the scene without feeling extremely fearful. You may use a pulse meter (Chapter 6) to monitor your body's performance.

1. Initial pulse reading (pulse meter) _____ (baseline)
2. You walk into the dental office _____ (pulse)
3. You are seated in the dental chair _____
4. The dentist enters the room _____
5. The dentist places a topical anesthetic cream on your gum to numb the injection site _____
6. The assistant hands the syringe to the dentist _____
7. The dentist places the syringe with the needle inside your mouth and begins to inject _____
8. You feel a slight pinch _____
9. During the injection, you feel a slight amount of pressure _____
10. The dentist finishes the injection _____
11. You now begin to feel numbness in your lip and cheek _____

Exercise No. 2. Again, visualize each scene, making sure to relax fully before proceeding onto the next scene.

1. You walk into the dental office _____
2. You are seated in the dental chair _____
3. The dentist enters the room _____
4. The dentist allows you to put on headphones and listen to your relaxation tape _____
5. The dentist positions the inhalation mask and allows you to breathe nitrous oxide to further relax _____
6. The dentist places a topical anesthetic cream on your gum _____
7. The dentist begins the injection of novocaine _____
8. You feel some pressure and a pinch _____

9. The injection is finished _____
10. You feel very proud of yourself _____

Exercise No. 3. Real-life application. (Do this only after you have mastered exercises 1 and 2).

1. Try to watch a dental or medical videotape showing an injection. See if your dentist has one. You might also try a medical or dental school if one is nearby. Consult the appendix for a list of dental fear treatment centers.
2. Ask your dentist whether you can hold a syringe and examine it. As you hold and examine it, practice deep relaxation until the fearful feelings go away. Take the cap off and note the small diameter of the needle. Dental needles are quite small compared to needles that are used to draw blood.
3. Imagine the needle, as you look at it, being placed inside your mouth. Imagine it penetrating and releasing the anesthetic solution. Imagine yourself successfully having this done.
4. When the dentist actually gives you an injection, if you still feel extremely apprehensive, you may decide to try the headphones, a relaxation tape, and nitrous oxide sedation.

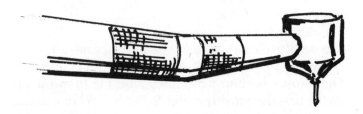

The Dental Drill

Fig. 13

DRILLING PHOBIA DESENSITIZATION

Exercise No. 1. Again try the imaginary method first. Look at a dental drill in Figure 13.

1. You walk into the dental office _____ (pulse)
2. You are seated in the dental chair _____
3. The dentist enters the room _____
4. The dentist offers you headphones, a relaxation tape, and nitrous oxide and you accept _____
5. You are becoming deeply relaxed _____
6. You are given an injection of novocaine _____
7. You can feel the profound effect of the numbness _____
8. After waiting several minutes, the dentist asks you how numb it feels and whether you are ready to proceed _____
9. The dentist begins to drill _____
10. As the noise of the drilling becomes louder, you increase the volume of your headphones _____
11. During the drilling, you feel a slight pressure in your tooth and a slight sensation of coldness _____
12. After the drilling, the dentist fills the tooth _____
13. At the completion of treatment, the dentist congratulates you for your excellent cooperation _____

Exercise No. 2.

1. Repeat exercise No. 1. Have an electric drill (such as a 3/8-inch Black and Decker) plugged in and ready to go.
2. When you reach scenes 9, 10, and 11, turn on the electric drill, increase the speed, and feel the vibrations, imagining the drill to be a dentist's drill in your mouth. *Do not put this drill near your mouth.*
3. Repeat this until your pulse remains near baseline during the exposure.

Exercise No. 3. Real-life application.

1. After your dentist has numbed you and is waiting for the numbness to work, ask whether you can look at and hold the drill. While you do this, become deeply relaxed.
2. Ask to hold the drill while the dentist turns it on. This can be an excellent way to desensitize your fear.
3. Ask whether the dentist will stop when you signal that you are in pain during the drilling.
4. After you successfully complete treatment, give yourself a reward for being good!

GAGGING PHOBIA DESENSITIZATION

Gagging during an impression (Figure 14) can be extremely uncomfortable and difficult to overcome. If you have only moderate success with this technique, you may wish to work with a professional therapist.

1. You walk into the dental office _____
2. You are seated in the dental chair _____
3. The dentist enters the room _____
4. The dentist offers you heaphones, the relaxation tape, and nitrous oxide sedation (nitrous oxide helps reduce gagging) _____
5. You become deeply relaxed _____
6. The dentist sits you upright in the dental chair _____
7. The dentist places an impression tray filled with a creamy material in your mouth _____
8. You can feel the cream touching the entire roof of your mouth _____
9. You may feel that the creamy material is pressing near the back of your throat _____
10. At this point, you feel like you might gag, but you resist the urge _____

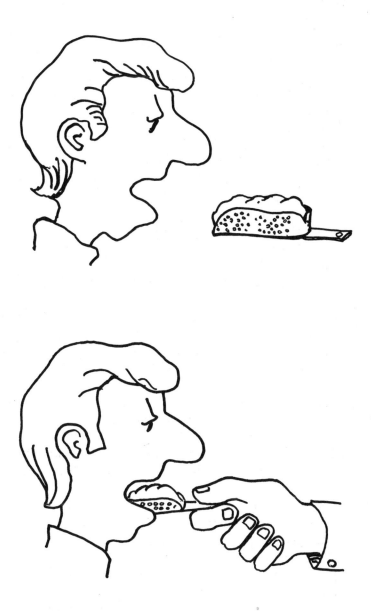

The Dental Impression

Fig. 14

11. After a few minutes, the dentist removes the tray with an excellent impression of your mouth and teeth _____

12. You feel confident you can go through that again _____

Exercise No. 2.

1. Repeat No. 1 exercise and, during scenes 7, 8, and 9, place a spoon on the roof of your mouth.
2. Slowly ease the spoon toward the back of your mouth until you feel a tendency to gag. Relax your tongue. Check your pulse.
3. Repeat this until you can place the spoon on the roof of the mouth near the last molars without gagging.
4. Practice breathing deeply through your nose during this exercise.
5. You can also practice lifting your leg halfway during the spoon exercise.
6. Researchers have found that some table salt applied to the tongue may help reduce gagging. Unless you are on a salt-restricted diet, place some salt on your tongue during this exercise.
7. The next time you need an impression, ask your dentist for any other suggestions that may help you.

DESENSITIZATION FOR FEAR
OF LACK OF CONTROL

This fear keeps many patients from returning to the dental office. Visualize the picture in Figure 15, which injects some humor into the concept that some patients have regarding this fear.

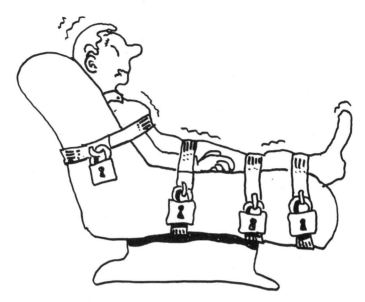

Lack of control in the dental chair

Fig. 15

Exercise No. 1. Visualize these scenes:

1. You are seated in the dental chair _____
2. The dentist enters the room _____
3. The dentist offers you nitrous oxide together with headphones and relaxation tapes _____
4. The dentist gives you an injection _____
5. After waiting, the dentist begins drilling on your tooth _____
6. During the drilling, you experience a sudden pain _____
7. At this, you raise your hand and the dentist stops the drilling _____
8. The dentist injects some more novocaine _____
9. The dentist continues drilling (no more pain) _____
10. The procedure is finished _____

Exercise No. 2. Real-life application.

1. When you visit your dentist for a procedure, discuss your concern about lack of control. Establish a signal so the dentist knows when you want to stop.
2. Remember that pain is always a possibility during dental treatment. The more *you* desensitize *yourself* and the more *you* raise *your* pain perception threshold, the more likely it is that *you will not feel pain* during dental procedures.

DESENSITIZATION FOR FEAR
OF EXTRACTION

Exercise No. 1. Years ago, you may have had a bad experience involving a difficult or painful extraction procedure. Today, teeth can be removed with efficient methods that allow the patient to be comfortable. Visualize these scenes:

1. You are seated in the dental chair _____
2. You meet the dentist _____
3. The dentist numbs your tooth to be extracted _____
4. After waiting for the numbness to become profound, the dentist begins to extract the tooth _____
5. You decide you would like nitrous oxide sedation, headphones, and a relaxation tape _____
6. After some time for relaxation, the dentist again begins

_____
7. You begin to feel some pressure on the tooth _____
8. You can hear some noise around the jawbone _____
9. After a few minutes, the dentist has extracted the tooth

_____
10. The dentist congratulates you for good cooperation

_____

CUSTOMIZED DESENSITIZATION
FOR YOUR INDIVIDUAL FEAR

To customize your own fear ladder, be creative. Start from the least provocative scene and progress to the most feared topic. Ask your dentist, a support person, or a therapist for help.

Your particular fear _____

Exercise No. 1: Construct your fear ladder.

Exercise No. 2: Add some element to mimic reality.

Exercise No. 3: Try to apply these methods to a real-life situation.

CONCLUSIONS ON DESENSITIZATION

1. To become successful with this technique, you must be able to become deeply relaxed. Check your skill with a pulse meter. In the dental office, you may choose headphones and nitrous oxide sedation to supplement your natural relaxation skills. Without deep relaxation, this method simply will not work.
2. Remember that the body cannot be relaxed and tense at the same time.
3. The more prolonged exposure (either mental or actual) to the feared stimulus, the better desensitization works.
4. Practice makes perfect — over and over and over again.

SELF-ASSESSMENT

1. My greatest fear(s) of dentistry is (are):

   _____

   _____

   _____

2. Who can be a support person for me? _____

3. How can I apply this to the "real" situation? _____

4. I can make a practice log. On a blank sheet of paper or a notebook:

Date	Time	Baseline Pulse	Highest Pulse

Keep track of your progress until your highest pulse during an exercise matches the baseline pulse.

12

PREVENTING DENTAL FEAR
IN CHILDREN

Many adults who have dental fear or dental phobia report that they have had bad childhood dental experiences. Many dental phobics claim that these experiences caused them to avoid dentistry for many years thereafter. Children are impressionable. Early life experiences often influence decisions made in adulthood. The purpose of this chapter is to help you insure that your children grow up with good memories of dentistry. Other books and pamphlets (such as those provided by the American Dental Association) give advice on proper dental care (brushing, flossing, diet, fluoride supplements) for children. Such advice is beyond the scope of this chapter.

Infants have certain "natural fears," such as fear of darkness, fear of falling, and fear of the unknown. One fear that infants don't have, however, is fear of dentists. Children enjoy going to the dentist today. In my practice, most of my patients who are children look forward to their semiannual checkup. Children acquire fear of the dentist from someone else or from a direct bad experience.

SOURCES OF FEAR IN CHILDREN

1. *The painful experience in a medical or dental office.* If your child has had a bad experience, he or she may instinctively resist going to the dentist. Some professional counseling may be in order. After a number of good experiences, the fear may decrease.

Recently, one of my adult fearful patients told me that when he was younger, his parents beat his brothers when they refused to go to the dentist. He decided to go to the dentist rather than be beaten. However, his dentist was so rough that he wished he had chosen the other alternative. The result was a lifetime of dental avoidance and a hostile attitude toward dentistry.

2. *By association with a previously acquired fear.* Children who have been injured and taken to a hospital may have experienced pain in connection with treatment for their injury. Hospitals usually have all white walls. Physicians and nurses are usually dressed in white from head to foot. When these children see white walls and white uniforms in a dental office, they may associate the dental office with the hospital and develop a fear reaction.
3. *By hearsay from friends, siblings, or other relatives.* Johnny likes his dentist. At his last checkup visit, he is told that he needs a filling. His parents, being very positive, do not make a big deal out of this. At school, however, one of his classmates tells him how awful it is to have a tooth filled and how much it hurts. At the appointment for the filling, the dentist and Johnny's parents cannot understand why Johnny is so afraid about this visit, until Johnny finally tells them about his classmate's scary story.

A few years ago, I conducted an informal survey about children's dental fears in second and third grades in several local schools. I was surprised to learn that even at this young age, a number of children had some fear of dentistry. In a lower socioeconomic school, more children reported dental fear than those in a higher socioeconomic school. This reaffirms an earlier research finding. This may suggest that the students in the former group had more decay (as the result of a high-sugar diet or improper oral hygiene), had acquired fear from hearsay of relatives or friends, or were treated (for economic reasons) in low-cost, high volume clinics. However, any parent, regardless of economic level, can prevent fear from developing in his or her child by following the pointers in this chapter.

THE CHILD'S FIRST VISIT TO THE DENTIST

Experts recommend that a child's first dental visit be by age one or two. This may seem a bit early, but there are several reasons. The major reason is preventing fear. The most important way of preventing fear is to let the child associate the dental office with happiness. If a child who has never been to the dentist has decay and develops a painful toothache at age three or four, the parent and the dentist have a difficult job. This may occur because some mothers put their babies to bed with a bottle of milk or a drink with sugar. The constant exposure of the teeth to sugar (milk has a sugar called lactose) often results in a condition called nursing bottle syndrome. The result can be extensive decay of many of the baby's teeth. It is better to fill the baby's bedtime bottle with plain water.

In many offices, children are introduced to dentistry in the "happy visit." In this visit, the child accompanies the parent or a sibling who is having his or her teeth checked and cleaned. The child observes the friendly and non-threatening interaction between patient and dentist. After one or two "happy visits," many children demand to have their turn in the dental chair. Their impression of dentistry begins on a positive note.

At this first checkup visit, the dentist and staff will stress the importance of prevention: good plaque control with brushing and flossing, proper nutrition, fluorides, and preventive sealants. Many children today have no decayed teeth as the result of prevention and semiannual checkups.

If the child needs a filling for a decayed tooth, several ideas can insure that the procedure goes well.

1. *Before the appointment.* Don't communicate your fears to your child. Some parents might say: "Johnny, don't worry about the filling; it probably won't hurt at all. Be a brave boy for Mommy and I'll give you a treat when you're finished." This type of statement will make the child feel that the dental experience *might* be a bad one. The bribe of offering a treat after the visit also makes the child wary of the procedure.

A better statement would be: "Johnny, we're going to the dentist's office today for your filling. The dentist will take care of your tooth and make it healthy again. When we're finished, we'll go for a treat." This matter-of-fact statement avoids the use of words such as hurt, bravery, pain, shots, needles, drilling. You can tell the child that you'll give him a treat afterward but don't make it contingent on good behavior during the appointment.

Schedule the appointment for the morning, if possible. Young children are rested then and are usually more cooperative than in the afternoon when they become tired.

Inform the dentist ahead of time about any particular needs your child might have: apprehension about the visit, medical problems, or other personal likes or dislikes. This gives the dentist the opportunity to plan the appointment to be as pleasant as possible.

2. *During the visit.* Follow your dentist's recommendation on whether you can accompany your child into the treatment room. Some offices allow the parent to sit quietly as

"a silent helper" in the treatment room while the child is treated. If you have extreme fear of dentistry, you probably should remain in the reception area. Your fearful behavior may be perceived by the child and may affect his behavior. Children can sense fearful signs such as sweaty body odor, tense muscles, strained voice. You may also put yourself through unnecessary anxiety by staying with the child.

3. *After the visit.* When the visit is over, praise your child for good behavior (if it was good) and give him a reward (preferably nothing with sugar). If the child's behavior was poor, don't praise it and don't give any reward. Rewarding poor performance merely encourages the child to repeat his poor behavior.

Be sure to follow the dentist's instructions about postoperative care. If a local anesthetic was used, you must closely monitor your child for lip, tongue, or cheek biting. Many children forget about this and can severely damage their lips or tongue. This can lead to fear of the dentist.

I once treated a young girl with a decayed tooth and used a small amount of local anesthetic to numb the area. The father was present during the appointment and heard our instructions about no roughhousing in order to avoid lip and tongue biting. Despite our warnings, the mother took the child to a festival, where the child jumped up and down in a large inflated balloon. Later the parents called me because the child's numb lip was cut severely. This caused considerable pain and required antibiotics and a long time to heal.

Such problems aside, from the dentist's standpoint, treating children can be one of the most rewarding aspects of dentistry. As Art Linkletter said, kids can say (and do) the darnedest things. Years ago, I treated a young girl, around age nine. I used conventional novocaine and completed two large fillings on moderately decayed upper molars. The procedure was fairly long, but the child behaved exceptionally well for her age. After the appointment, the child drew the picture shown below.

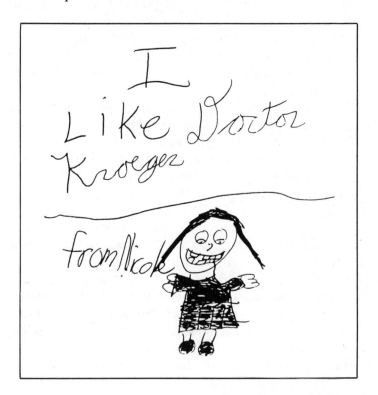

TEENAGERS

Teenagers fall into the awkward category between childhood and adulthood. Many teenagers resent authority figures. To be successful with these patients, the dentist must learn to communicate as a friend and not as an authority figure. Some teenagers are fearful because they were hurt by a dentist in childhood. In this situation, the dentist must uncover the fears and be very gentle, realizing that the teenager may be under considerable stress from outside (peer pressure) or inside influences (the growing-up process) in addition to fear of dentistry.

WHAT THE DENTIST CAN DO

The dentist can provide many things to make the dental visit for the child a positive one:

- friendly office staff
- a children's corner with games
- a video game for distraction
- asking the child for his or her help
- a bulletin board with pictures of "Super Patients"
- being gentle and taking extra time, if needed

Some children who are fearful or uncooperative may require medication before the appointment to make them sleepy. Some very young children with extensive decay may require a general anesthetic in a hospital.

Because children often take more time for their treatment than adults, their fees may be as high or higher than fees for adults. The dentist's objective is to deliver a high-quality dental restoration on a relaxed patient in a gentle manner. Most parents want nothing but the best for their children. To accomplish this, the dentist must take time and have patience.

A SUMMARY OF DO'S AND DON'TS

DON'T:

- tell your child about all your dental fears
- use bribery
- wait until your child has a toothache before introducing him or her to the dentist
- use fear-producing words such as: pain, bravery, hurt, etc.
- worry if your child doesn't behave perfectly; this may not be a reflection on your child-rearing.

DO:

- tell your child to ignore any scary stories about the dentist from friends or in the media
- speak in positive terms about the dentist
- read a book about the dentist to your child
- make the dental visit a fun experience
- be honest with your child about his or her questions. Don't promise him the moon.
- make the appointment in the morning
- take your child for semiannual dental checkups
- set a good example by brushing, flossing, and maintaining good nutrition. Children learn good or bad habits from their parents.

By using these concepts, you and your child can enjoy your dental visits and prevent fear from developing. Having a good, gentle dentist is also important, as the next chapter shows.

13

SELECTING A GENTLE DENTIST AND STAFF

Many patients who have been hurt in a dental office doubt that they can find a gentle dentist who will take time and be considerate of them and their fears. However, today most dentists are very gentle and willing to take extra time to listen to the fearful dental patient. How then can the fearful patient select a dentist who excels both in the technical and the human side of dentistry?

First, quality in the mind of the patient differs from quality in the mind of the dentist. The dentist views quality in terms of technical excellence: a bite harmonious with the teeth and jaw joint, fine margins on a crown, healthy supporting gum and bones. The patient views quality in terms of chewing ability, good-looking teeth, and a comfortable mouth. The patient cannot evaluate the margins of a crown (cap) or measure a gum pocket. The patient can, however, evaluate other variables: the dentist being on time, respecting the patient, not criticizing the patient, and being gentle.

In choosing dental services, most people want the highest quality for the lowest price. To want this is human nature.

Therefore, most people will shop for the best price for a certain item. Most people know that good quality isn't cheap. Good quality may outlive a cheaper price. Someone once said, "Quality is never an accident, it is always the result of high intention, sincere effort, intelligent direction, and skillful execution: it represents the wise choice of many masters." Therefore, the lowest-priced dentist may not be able to offer the best quality dental treatment. Most fearful patients would prefer a quality dental restoration *compared to one that will need replacing a few years hence.* To a fearful patient, quality means, most important, the dentist being gentle and taking time. Conversely, the most expensive dentist may not deliver the highest quality care. You, the patient, must judge for yourself. Several parameters in this chapter will help you.

The goal for the fearful patient is to develop a relationship of friendship with the dentist and staff. Does the dentist seem *genuinely* interested in you as a person? Do the dentist and staff seem honest to you? Do they have character and integrity? These are important considerations for you. Do you want someone without integrity to be working inside your mouth?

SELECTION PROCESS

1. *Finding a dentist to call for your first appointment.* This may be difficult, especially if you have recently moved to a new city.

   - Ask trusted friends or relatives if they know of a gentle dentist. Describe your fears and concerns.
   - Call the local dental society (a chapter of the American Dental Association). Ask them to recommend a dentist who has special interest in dental phobics. Describe your fears and concerns.
   - Contact a local dental fear treatment center if one exists in

your area. See the Appendix for a list of such centers.

- Ask your family physician. If you are a dental phobic, your physician may be able to suggest a counselor to help you prepare for your dental visit.
- Ask a periodontist (gum specialist, listed in the yellow pages). This specialist usually sees patients from a variety of general dentists and knows which dentists do excellent technical dental work.
- Dentists who advertise to perform gentle dentistry may indeed be sincere in this promise. But, if you feel that you are not being treated gently enough, the dentist is not living up to the advertisement. Choose again. An old saying goes: "Beware of bargains in parachutes, brain surgery, and dental care."
- Certain dental insurance programs are designed to move a large volume of patients in and out of the dental office. Be cautious about such programs if you think you are not being treated as an individual. Every patient has this right.

2. *The initial phone call.* You now have the name of a recommended dentist to call. You have decided to make an appointment. What should you look for in the initial phone conversation?

- Note the sound of the receptionist's voice. Does she sound happy or worried or overworked or blah?
- Express your fears and concerns. Ask whether the dentist is interested in treating fearful patients. Does he or she have any kind of a dental fear control program? Is nitrous oxide available? What can he do for your specific fears?
- Does the receptionist seem truly interested in you?

3. *You arrive at the dental office.* What can you tell about quality of dental service by the exterior or interior of the office?

- Is the parking lot clean or littered excessively?
- Is the exterior of the office neat or is paint peeling or are there other signs of disrepair?
- Is the interior of the office quiet, peaceful, and well-decorated? Does the office seem to be organized? Is it neat and clean? Do you smell an offensive odor? Does the office atmosphere seem calm and relaxing to you?

4. *You are greeted by the receptionist.* Does she use your name? Does she convey a feeling of warmth and caring?
5. *You meet the dentist and assistant.* This may or may not be for actual treatment.

- Are they neat, clean, and organized? Does the dentist respect the staff? Do they seem happy?
- Do they appear healthy and health-oriented? What do their teeth look like? Recently, a patient told me that his wife and children did not like their former dentist because he always smelled from cigarette smoke, and his treatment was rough.

6. *Actual treatment begins.* Although every treatment is different, these guidelines should apply almost universally.

- Communicate your fears and concerns about the procedure to the dentist and staff.
- Have a signal (such as raising your hand) to let the dentist know if you are in pain or if you want to rest or stop. You may want to rinse or take a stretch break. Remember that the dentist can only do so much. You must accept responsibility to learn relaxation exercises. However, if the dentist does not stop when you are in pain, you have the right to get out of the chair. *You do not have to let the dentist hurt you.* If the dentist tells you the drilling will continue for only a few more seconds, try to have patience. He or she is trying to do a good job by removing all the decay or finishing the procedure correctly. If the "few seconds"

turns into 15 or 30 seconds or a few minutes, this is unnecessary. You do not have to be a martyr and endure this pain. Techniques are available in dentistry to stop this kind of discomfort during drilling. By using the periodontal ligament injection, the dentist can usually eliminate all pain during the drilling. As with anything, there are exceptions to this rule.

- The dentist should avoid whatever it is you do not like, if possible. If you don't like hearing about the procedure in detail, explain this to the dentist. Some patients become faint or nauseated when some procedures are described in detail.
- If you do not like some necessary aspect of the procedure (such as the impression of your mouth), explain this to the dentist. Any feared, but necessary, procedure should be introduced slowly and gently.
- Anytime the dentist or staff causes you pain, they should stop immediately. They should then give you the option of having additional novocaine for pain control.
- Many patients play a passive role in their dental treatment. Be assertive! If there is something you don't like, say so. Most dentists want to keep you as a patient and they are more than willing to help you get through the procedure. If you don't perceive the dentist and staff to be helpful and considerate, switch dentists.

7. *The treatment is finished.* Decide whether this was a good experience or a bad one. Even gentle dentists can't be all things to all people. You may want to consider giving your dentist a second chance before choosing another dentist.

- Do you need additional counseling for your fear — such as a dental fear control program or a mental health specialist?
- Remember that uncontrolled fear will result in more dental problems for you and usually a higher cost.

- Another key factor in selecting a dentist is whether he or she is prevention-oriented. If the dentist tells you that you must have all your teeth extracted and wear dentures, you may want to first consult with a periodontist. A periodontist can save teeth that seem to be hopeless because of gum problems. Many phobic patients I have seen have extensive decay and gum disease. Occasionally, a patient may need full mouth extractions. Usually, though, teeth can be saved and restored beautifully for a lifetime of function and enjoyment.

Finally, do the dentist and staff seem *genuinely* interested in your overall health as well as in your dental health? Are you just a number in their system? Do you merely represent x amount of dollars to be produced next month? Or are you a person whom the dentist and staff sincerely want to help reach optimal oral health, which will in turn contribute to an increased level of health and wellness?

SELF-ASSESSMENT

1. How will I proceed to locate a gentle dentist?

   - asks friends or relatives
   - call the local dental society
   - call the closest dental college

2. When will I do this?

3. What are the things I will expect to find in the dental office?

   _____

   _____

   _____

   _____

4. How will I best establish rapport with my new dentist?

   _____

   _____

14

NOW, YOU'RE READY TO GO

These comments may help you make and keep that first appointment or improve your relationship with your current dentist.

1. *Appointments / cancellations.*

Before you make your appointment (especially if you have not seen a dentist in many years and whether you have extreme fear), decide whether you need outside help. Should you have counseling with a psychotherapist before the dental appointment? Should a support person accompany you to the office? Should your first office visit be one where you tour the office and meet the dentist or go through the dental fear control program? This is an important decision, because some dental phobics make an appointment and then, on the day of the appointment, overwhelmed by fear, cancel or miss the appointment. This is very frustrating for the dentist and staff who have reserved the appointment time. Since they cannot fill a last minute cancellation or a failed appointment slot, they are actually losing money, which increases their overhead. These are the people who are trying to help you. Be nice to them: Don't fail appointments and, if you absolutely have to cancel the appointment, give at least 48 hours' notice.

If canceling or missing appointments (because of fear) becomes a habit for you, you may need counseling or a support person to help you keep your appointments. Some dental phobics unknowingly suffer from "counterphobic repetition," where they repeatedly schedule and cancel their dental appointments without realizing that their phobia is the underlying cause of their habitual canceling behavior.

Most dental offices simply cannot afford to treat a patient who continually cancels or misses appointments. Usually this cost is passed on to the patient who cancels. Often, the office will dismiss the patient and recommend that the patient find a new dentist.

2. *Make the appointment now. Don't wait till it hurts!*

Many dental phobics treat their own dental maladies, even if they are in pain, rather than face the dentist. However, this can backfire and cause serious medical complications. Recently, a dental phobic died because of an uncontrolled infection that originated in his mouth and spread throughout his system. Sometimes we find oral cancer in the mouth. This too can spread throughout the body if it is not treated in an early stage.

Delaying treatment usually means the cost of treatment will increase. If a small cavity is repaired in a tooth, the cost is much less than the cost of root canal therapy that would be required if the cavity, untreated for a prolonged time, spread into the nerve of the tooth.

Postponing treatment also usually means the treatment will take longer, be more complex, and possibly more upsetting for you. Be kind to yourself — make your appointment now before you have a dental emergency.

3. *Communication with the dentist and staff.*

The best way to achieve a good, trusting relationship with the dentist is through effective communication. You must learn to be assertive enough to get your point across to the dentist. If you don't express all your fears or concerns, he or she may do something you don't like. Likewise, the dentist must communicate well with you.

If you do have a misunderstanding with the dentist or with one of the staff, try to understand that it may be a communication problem. Try your best to work out a solution. Most problems can be solved by mutual discussion.

4. *Your treatment may be substantial.*

If you have avoided the dentist for a long period of time, your treatment may be complex and time-consuming. Your mouth did not deteriorate overnight. Accordingly, your treatment will require careful planning and dedication to detail by your dentist. The fee for your treatment may or may not be considerable. If you have not visited the dentist in many years, prepare yourself for "sticker shock."

Consider the concept of value versus need. A need is a necessity or an obligation. When a person is told he or she needs something, he may resent the need. When a person is told he needs something, he is often highly concerned about the cost. If a person knows he needs extensive dental treatment, he may resent that need and dread having the work completed. Value is relative worth or importance: the degree of excellence. When people value something, they sincerely have a strong desire for that something.

Dentists want to know *your needs, your desires, and your values.* We want to know what your oral health and your teeth mean to you in terms of value. Henry Ford once said,

"He who needs an article, and does without it, pays for it whether he buys it or not." Learn to value excellent dentistry. It is well worth the investment. You have suffered with fear for a long time. Choose an excellent dentist who will perform treatment that will last you many, many years.

5. *Have patience with the progress of your treatment.*

Now that your burden of fear has been lifted, you may feel that you want your mouth restored as quickly as possible. This is a natural human reaction. But please have patience. Your dentist, in order to accomplish excellent dentistry, may design a treatment plan that may require considerable time. Other specialists may need to be consulted in the planning phases and they may actually perform some of the treatment. Remember your goal: to have a healthy mouth and beautiful smile. Go easy on your dentist: he's trying to do his best. Don't strap him with time limits and other pressure tactics.

6. *Learning to trust the dental team.*

Many dental phobics find it difficult to place themselves in a passive, reclined position in the dental chair and then to *trust* the dentist, who represents potential pain and suffering. Trust is essential to this relationship. You have to work at developing it. The dentist also must earn your trust.

Learning to be friends with the dentist is also difficult for fearful patients. However, this type of relationship allows the dentist to help the patient to good oral health.

THE DAY OF YOUR FIRST APPOINTMENT

On the day of your appointment, don't eat or drink anything with caffeine. Avoid nicotine. These will stimulate you and make you agitated. Even such drinks as cocoa and decaffeinated coffee have some caffeine.

Eat something with protein or carbohydrate about one hour before your visit. This will reduce the possiblity of being irritable due to hunger and will reduce the chance of fainting due to low blood sugar.

Practice relaxation about one hour before your appointment. Use either progressive muscle relaxation or guided imagery or another method that you prefer. Information on purchasing a relaxation training audiocassette is given in the Appendix. Become as deeply relaxed as you can. Practice this all the way to the office (use caution if you are driving), in the reception area, and in the treatment room.

Use "thought stoppage": If negative thoughts such as memories of bad experiences or canceling enter your mind, drive them out. Don't let them hurt you. Use positive thoughts and positive self-talk continually. Tell yourself that you can do it.

When you arrive in the dental office, bring your headphones and your relaxation tape. If you have to wait for a considerable amount of time, you can listen to the tapes to relax yourself. When you meet the staff, ask for a tour of the office. This will help dispel the fear of the unknown that many fearful patients have.

When you meet the dentist, discuss your fears and your concerns honestly and openly. Ask the dentist for suggestions. Describe your ideas and strategies for coping with the fears. This initial interview will allow you to get to know your dentist and vice versa. Remember: Getting your fears out in the open is half the battle.

In our office, we do one of the following at the initial appointment for the fearful patient:

- dental fear control program
- initial examination including any necessary x-rays

Ask your dentist about other methods to help you to have

your dental treatment completed comfortably. If you have the initial examination and do not want to hear the results, tell your dentist. You may defer hearing this to a future appointment.

At the end of this appointment, you will make another appointment. This may be for a consultation or a simple procedure to build your confidence such as a prophylaxis (cleaning and polishing of the teeth).

After the successful appointment, congratulate yourself and treat yourself and your support person to a surprise. After all, you deserve it!

I hope this book has helped you to reduce your fear or to find a gentle dentist or psychotherapist to help you. To overcome a phobia is not particularly easy. It requires firm dedication and hard, hard work. Put your goal of a healthy mouth and beautiful smile on paper and list a plan of action. Then carry it out to completion. If you are successful in overcoming your dental fear, I'd like to hear about it and would appreciate your letters. Please send them to the publisher's (Heritage Communications) address in the front of this book. Conversely, if you have a problem you can't seem to resolve, I'd also be interested in hearing about that. As someone once said, "Success comes in cans, not in can'ts." Good luck and I wish you well!

SELF-ASSESSMENT

1. How did I do with this book? _____

2. Who is my support person? _____

3. My chief fears to present to my dentist are:

   _____

   _____

   _____

4. Goals for my first appointment:

   - _____

   - _____

   - _____

5. The date for my first appointment: _____
   - My commitment to follow through with this appointment is:
     (circle one)   excellent   good   maybe   poor

   - I will be on time for my appointment and I will have a positive mental attitude.

APPENDIX

AUDIOCASSETTE ON
RELAXATION TRAINING

This tape, *Learning the Relaxation Response,* features the voice of Dr. Kroeger and has been used by many of his dental phobic patients, 98 percent of whom found the tape to help them reduce their dental fear. On side A, training in progressive muscle relaxation enables the listener to achieve a profound state of calmness by totally relaxing all the muscles in the body. On side B, the listener is trained in guided imagery and learns to imagine and focus on several relaxation-inducing scenes. Peaceful music and other relaxing effects are woven into this tape.

This tape is designed specifically for the fearful or phobic dental patient. Other relaxation tapes are available through various sources that may also help.

To order a copy of this tape, please write or call:

Heritage Communications
11469 Lippelman Rd.
Cincinnati, Ohio 45246
Phone (513) 771-2230

Another tape program on overcoming dental fear is called *Overcoming Your Fear of the Dentist* by Dr. Leonard G. Horowitz. It is available by writing:

Tetrahedron, Inc.
P.O. Box 402
Rockport, Mass. 01966

DENTAL FEAR TREATMENT CENTERS

The following centers are dedicated to treating fearful dental patients. These centers are associated with dental schools and hospitals and usually bring together a team of professionals to help the dental phobic to optimum oral health.

WEST

Dental Fears Treatment Clinic, School of Dentistry, University of Washington, Seattle, Washington.

Dental Fears Center, Mount Zion Hospital, San Francisco, California.

MIDWEST

Dental Fears Clinic, College of Dentistry, University of Kentucky, Lexington, Kentucky.

Dental Fear Clinic, Evanston Hospital (Northwestern University), 2650 Ridge Ave., Evanston, Illinois.

SOUTH

Dental Behavioral Research Clinic, Florida State University, Talahassee, Florida.

College of Dentistry, University of Florida, Gainesville, Florida.

Eastern Carolina University, Dental Fear Clinic, Family Medicine, Greenville, North Carolina.

EAST

Dental Phobia Clinic, Mount Sinai Medical Center, New York City, New York.

Dental Fear Clinic, Department of Dentistry, The Medical Center of Delaware, Wilmington Hospital, Wilmington, Delaware.

Please Note: If you can't get to one of these centers, they may be able to refer you to a dentist in your area. Many of these centers keep lists of dentists who have taken their courses in treating fearful patients.

BIBLIOGRAPHY AND
SUGGESTED READINGS

Although most of the following references are taken from the scientific literature, some of the books listed below may give you additional insight into natural relaxation methods and ways to cope with fear.

BOOKS

Benson, H. *The Relaxation Response*. New York: Avon Books, 1976.

Caprio, F. S. and Berger, J. R. *Helping Yourself with Self-Hypnosis*. New York: Warner Books, 1968.

Christensen, G. *Clinical Research Associates Newsletter* 9 (1985): 1-3.

Fensterheim, H., and Baer, J. *Stop Running Scared*. New York: Dell, 1978.

Green, M. *Living Fear Free*. New York: Warner Books, 1987.

Ingersoll, B. D. *Behavioral Aspects in Dentistry*. New York: Appleton-Century-Crofts, 1982.

Jacobson, E. *Progressive Relaxation*. Chicago: University of Chicago Press, 1938.

Kroeger, R. F. *Managing the Apprehensive Dental Patient*. Cincinnati: Heritage Communications, 1987.

Le Cron, L. M. *Self Hypnotism*. New York: New American Library, 1970.

Mavissakalian, M. and Barlow, D.H., eds. *Phobia: Psychological and Pharmacological Treatment.* New York: Guilford Press, 1981.

Malamed, S. *Sedation: A Guide to Patient Management.* St. Louis: C.V. Mosby Co., 1985.

Melzack, R. and Wall, P. D. *The Challenge of Pain.* New York: Basic Books, 1982.

Milgrom, P., et al. *Treating Fearful Dental Patients.* Reston, Va.: Reston Publishing Co., 1985.

Rugh, J. D. et al., eds. *Biofeedback in Dentistry: Research and Clinical Applications.* Phoenix, Az.: Semantodontics, 1977.

Trieger, N. *Pain Control.* Chicago: Quintessence Books, 1974.

Wenrich, W. W., et al. *Self-directed Systematic Desensitization.* Bridgewater, N.J.: F. Fournies and Associates, Inc., 1976.

Wolpe, J. *Psychotherapy by Reciprocal Inhibition.* Stanford, Calif.: Stanford University Press, 1958.

JOURNALS

Carlsson, S. G. et al. "Reduction of tension in fearful dental patients." *Journal of the American Dental Association* 101 (1980): 638-641.

Corah, N. L. "Development of a dental anxiety scale." *Journal of Dental Research* 48 (1969): 596.

Corah, N. L. et al. "The use of relaxation and distraction to reduce psychological stress during dental procedures." *Journal of the American Dental Association* 98 (1979): 390-394.

Gale, E. N., and Ayer, W.A. "Treatment of dental phobias." *Journal of the American Dental Association* 78 (1969): 1304.

Gatchel, R. J., et al. "The prevalence of dental fear and avoidance: a recent survey study." *Journal of the American Dental Association* 107 (1983): 609-610.

Hawley, B. P., et al. "The first dental visit for children from low socioeconomic families." *Journal of Dentistry for Children* 41 (1974): 376-381.

Hirschman, R. "Physiological feedback and stress reduction." In "Behavioral Approaches to Dental Fear, Pain, and Stress," symposium presented at the meeting of the Society of Behavioral Medicine, New York, 1980.

Jackson, E. "Managing dental fears: A treatment code of practice." *Journal of Oral Medicine* 29 (1974): 96-101.

Kaufman, E. et al. "Difficulties in achieving local anesthesia." *Journal of the American Dental Association* 108 (1984): 205-208.

Kleinknecht, R. A., et al. "Factor analysis of the Dental Fear Survey with cross validation." *Journal of the American Dental Association* 108 (1984): 59-61.

Kleinknecht, R. A., et al. "Origins and characteristics of fear of dentistry." *Journal of the American Dental Association* 86 (1973): 842-848.

Klepac, R. K. "Successful treatment of avoidance of dentistry by desensitization or by increasing pain tolerance." *Journal of Behavioral Therapy and Experimental Psychology* 6 (1975): 307.

Kroeger, R. F. "Help patients overcome dental fear." *Dental Economics* 75 (1985): 40-45.

Kroeger, R. F. "Levels of fear or phobia and a formal dental fear control program." *General Dentistry* 34 (1986):241-242.

Kroeger, R. F. "Management of dental phobia: the use of fear-screening questionnaires." *International Journal of Psychosomatics* 33 (1986): 92-95.

Kroeger, R. F. "The dental fear control program: a behavioral model to treat dental phobia." *Journal of the Massachusetts Dental Society* 35 (1986): 175-180.

Melamed, B. G., et al. "Reduction of fear-related dental management problems with use of filmed modeling." *Journal of the American Dental Association* 90 (1975): 822-825.

Scott, D. S., et al. "Historical antecedents of dental anxiety." *Journal of the American Dental Association* 108 (1984): 42-45.

Scott, D. S., and Hirschman, R. "Psychological aspects of dental anxiety in adults." *Journal of the American Dental Association* 104 (1982): 27-31.

Seeman, K., and Molin, C. "Psychopathology, feelings of confinement and helplessness in the dental chair, and the relationship of the dentist in patients with disproportionate dental anxiety (DDA)." *ACTA Psychiatra Scandinavica* 54 (1976): 81-91.

Shaw, D. W., and Thoresen, C. E. "Effects of modeling and desensitization in reducing dentist phobia." *Journal of Counseling Psychology* 21 (1974): 415-420.

Smith, T., et al. "An evaluation of an institution-based dental fears clinic." *Journal of Dental Research* 63 (1984): 272.

Walton, R. E., and Abbott, B. J. "Periodontal ligament injection: a clinical evaluation." *Journal of the American Dental Association* 103 (1981): 571-575.

Weinstein, P., et al. "The effect of dentists' behaviors on fear-related behaviors in children." *Journal of the American Dental Association* 104 (1982): 32-38.

ABOUT THE AUTHOR

Dr. Kroeger is a full-time general dentist practicing in Cincinnati. In addition to being a guest lecturer at the University of Kentucky's College of Dentistry, he treats many fearful and phobic patients in his private practice. He is the originator of the dental fear control program, a self-help, non-drug approach to conquering fear of dentistry. This program has been nationally recognized by the American Fund for Dental Health through a generous research grant to the University of Kentucky. In this grant, dental offices in four states are being trained to conduct the dental fear control program for their patients. Dr. Kroeger serves as the principal consultant to this project. Dr. Kroeger has written numerous articles for dental journals and magazines on the topic of dental fear management. He is the author of *Managing the Apprehensive Dental Patient,* a text for dentists and their staffs. This book was featured as a selection in Semantodontics' Book-of-the-Month Club. Dr. Kroeger has given numerous seminars on these topics in this country and abroad.